# Advanced Life Support

## 5th Edition

ISBN 1-903812-11-9
April 2006

ADVANCED LIFE SUPPORT

ALS

i

# Advanced Life Support
## 5th Edition

## Editorial Board

Jerry Nolan (Chairman)

Jasmeet Soar

Andy Lockey

David Pitcher

David Gabbott

Gavin Perkins

Mike Scott

Sarah Mitchell

## Contributors

Gamal Abbas

Annette Alfonzo

Hans-Richard Arntz

Alessandro Barelli

Peter Baskett

Leo Bossaert

Charles Deakin

Patrick Druwé

David Gabbott

Sarah Gill

Max Groenhart

Carl Gwinnutt

Anthony Handley

Bob Harris

Sara Harris

Freddy Lippert

Andy Lockey

David Lockey

Carsten Lott

Oliver Meyer

Sarah Mitchell

Koen Monsieurs

Jerry Nolan

Gavin Perkins

David Pitcher

Maureen Ryan

Claudio Sandroni

Mike Scott

Gary Smith

Jasmeet Soar

Karl Thies

## Acknowledgements

We thank Mike Scott for his dual talents as photographer and ALS instructor – he has shot and digitally prepared all the photographs in this manual. We also thank Oliver Meyer for digital preparation of the all the 12-lead ECGs and rhythm strips, Correen Cleggett for help with the final preparation for printing, and the models for their help with the photographs.

Published by Resuscitation Council (UK)

5th Floor, Tavistock House North, Tavistock Square, London WC1H 9HR

Tel: 020 7388 4678   Fax: 020 7383 0773   E-mail: enquiries@resus.org.uk   Website: http://www.resus.org.uk

Printed by: TT Litho Printers Limited

Corporation Street, Rochester, Kent. ME1 1NN

Tel: 01634 845397   Fax: 01634 846807   Email: admin@ttlitho.co.uk   Website: http://www.ttlitho.co.uk

# Contents

# Glossary

Throughout this publication:

- The masculine pronouns he, him and his are used generically.
- The terms cardiopulmonary arrest, cardiorespiratory arrest and cardiac arrest have been used interchangeably.
- Adrenaline is the preferred term for adrenaline/epinephrine.

| | |
|---|---|
| AC | alternating current |
| ACEI | angiotensin converting enzyme inhibitor |
| ACS | acute coronary syndrome |
| AED | automated external defibrillator |
| AF | atrial fibrillation |
| ALS | advanced life support |
| AMI | acute myocardial infarction |
| AV | atrioventricular as in atrioventricular node |
| AVNRT | AV nodal re-entry tachyarrhythmia |
| AVRT | AV re-entry tachyarrhythmia |
| BLS | basic life support- no equipment is used except protective devices |
| BP | blood pressure |
| CCU | coronary care unit |
| CK | creatine kinase |
| CHB | complete heart block |
| CPR | cardiopulmonary resuscitation - refers to chest compressions and ventilations |
| CVP | central venous pressure |
| DC | direct current |
| DNAR | do not attempt resuscitation |
| ECG | electrocardiogram |
| ED | emergency department |
| EMS | emergency medical services, e.g., ambulance service |
| HDU | high dependence unit |
| ICD | implantable cardioverter-defibrillator |
| ICU | intensive care unit |
| IM | intramuscular |
| IO | intraosseous |
| IV | intravenous |
| JVP | jugular venous pressure |
| Lidocaine | the preferred term for lignocaine |
| LMA | laryngeal mask airway |
| LT | Laryngeal Tube |
| LV | left ventricular |
| MET | medical emergency team |
| MILS | manual in-line stabilisation |
| NSTEMI | non-ST elevation myocardial infarction |
| PCI | percutaneous intervention |
| PEA | pulseless electrical activity |
| PLMA | ProSeal LMA |
| ROSC | return of spontaneous circulation |
| RV | right ventricular |
| SA | sino-atrial as in sino-atrial node |
| SBP | systolic blood pressure |
| STEMI | ST elevation myocardial infarction |
| SVT | supraventricular tachycardia |
| VF | ventricular fibrillation |
| VT | ventricular tachycardia |
| VF/VT | VF/pulseless VT |
| WPW | Wolff-Parkinson-White syndrome |

ALS

# Advanced Life Support in Perspective

## CHAPTER 1

## Introduction: the problem

Ischaemic heart disease is the leading cause of death in the world. In Europe, cardiovascular disease accounts for around 40% of all deaths under the age of 75 years. Sudden cardiac arrest is responsible for more than 60% of adult deaths from coronary heart disease. Summary data from 37 communities in Europe indicate that the annual incidence of emergency medical services (EMS)-treated out-of-hospital cardiorespiratory arrests for all rhythms is 38 per 100,000 population. Based on these data, the annual incidence of ventricular fibrillation (VF) arrest is 17 per 100,000. Survival to hospital discharge is 10.7% for all-rhythm cardiac arrest and 21.2% for VF cardiac arrest.

One third of all people developing a myocardial infarction die before reaching hospital; most of them die within an hour of the onset of acute symptoms. In most of these deaths the presenting rhythm is VF or pulseless ventricular tachycardia (VF/VT). The only effective treatment for these arrhythmias is attempted defibrillation, and with each minute's delay the chances of a successful outcome fall by about 7-10%. Once the patient is admitted to hospital the incidence of VF after myocardial infarction is approximately 5%.

The incidence of in-hospital cardiac arrest is difficult to assess because it is influenced heavily by factors such as the criteria for hospital admission and implementation of a do-not-attempt-resuscitation (DNAR) policy. The incidence of primary cardiac arrest in hospital is approximately 1.5-3.0/1000 admissions. In about two thirds of in-hospital cardiac arrests the first monitored rhythm is non-VF/VT (asystole or pulseless electrical activity (PEA)). Many of these patients have significant comorbidity, which influences the initial rhythm and, in these cases, strategies to prevent cardiac arrest are particularly important.

## The Chain of Survival

The interventions that contribute to a successful outcome after a cardiac arrest can be conceptualised as a chain - the Chain of Survival (Figure 1.1).

The chain is only as strong as its weakest link; all four links of the Chain of Survival must be strong. They are:

- early recognition and call for help;
- early cardiopulmonary resuscitation (CPR);
- early defibrillation;
- post-resuscitation care.

## Early recognition and call for help

Out of hospital, early recognition of the importance of chest pain will enable the victim or a bystander to call the EMS and receive treatment that may prevent cardiac arrest. After out-of-hospital cardiac arrest, immediate access to the EMS is vital. In most countries access to the EMS is achieved by means of a single telephone number.

In-hospital, early recognition of the critically ill patient who is at risk of cardiac arrest and a call for the resuscitation team or medical emergency team (MET) will enable treatment to prevent cardiac arrest (Chapter 2). A universal number for calling the resuscitation team or MET should be adopted in all hospitals. If cardiac arrest occurs, do not delay defibrillation until arrival of the resuscitation team — clinical staff should be trained to use a defibrillator.

## Early CPR

Chest compressions and ventilation of the victim's lungs will slow down the rate of deterioration of the brain and heart. After out-of-hospital cardiac arrest, bystander CPR extends the period for successful resuscitation and probably doubles the chance of survival. Despite this fact, in most European countries bystander CPR is carried out in only a minority of cases. After in-hospital cardiac arrest, chest compressions and ventilation must be undertaken immediately, but should not delay attempts to defibrillate those patients in VF/VT. Interruptions to chest compressions must be minimised and should occur only briefly during defibrillation attempts and rhythm checks.

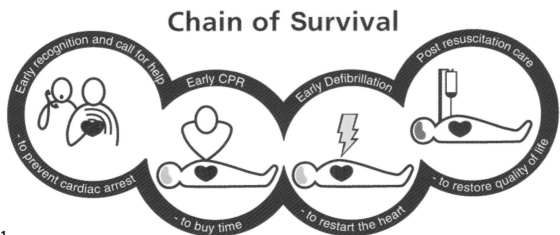

**Figure 1.1**

## Early defibrillation

After out-of-hospital cardiac arrest, the goal is to deliver a shock (if indicated) within 5 min of the EMS receiving the call. In many areas achievement of this goal will require the introduction of Public Access Defibrillation (PAD) programs using automated external defibrillators (AEDs). In hospitals, sufficient healthcare personnel should be trained and authorised to use a defibrillator to enable the first responder to a cardiac arrest to attempt defibrillation when indicated, without delay, in virtually every case.

## Post-resuscitation care

Return of a spontaneous circulation (ROSC) is an important phase in the continuum of resuscitation; however, the ultimate goal is to return the patient to a state of normal cerebral function, a stable cardiac rhythm, and normal haemodynamic function, so that they can leave hospital in reasonable health at minimum risk of a further cardiac arrest. The quality of advanced life support (ALS) in the post-resuscitation period influences the patient's ultimate outcome. The post-resuscitation phase starts at the location where ROSC is achieved. The ALS provider must be capable of providing high quality post-resuscitation care until the patient is transferred to an appropriate high-care area.

## Science and guidelines

The publication of the 2005 International Consensus on Cardiopulmonary Resuscitation and Emergency Cardiovascular Care Science with Treatment Recommendations was the culmination of a prolonged period of collaboration between resuscitation experts from around the world. The European Resuscitation Council (ERC) Guidelines for Resuscitation 2005 are derived from this consensus document and the contents of this ALS provider manual are consistent with these guidelines. Most resuscitation organisations in Europe have ratified and adopted the ERC guidelines.

## ALS algorithm

The ALS algorithm (Figure 1.2) is the centre point of the ALS course and is applicable to most cardiopulmonary resuscitation situations. Some modifications may be required when managing cardiac arrest in special circumstances (Chapter 13).

## The ALS course

The ALS course provides a standardised approach to cardiopulmonary resuscitation in adults. The course is targeted at doctors, nurses, and other healthcare professionals who are expected to provide ALS in and out of hospital. The multidisciplinary nature of the course encourages efficient teamwork. By training together, all ALS providers are given the opportunity to gain experience as both resuscitation team members and team leaders.

The course comprises workshops, skill stations, cardiac arrest simulation (CAS) training, and lectures. Candidates' knowledge is assessed by means of a multiple choice question paper. Practical skills in airway management and the initial approach to a collapsed patient (including defibrillation where appropriate) are assessed continuously. There is also assessment of a simulated cardiac arrest (CASTest). Candidates reaching the required standard receive an ALS provider certificate. It has been demonstrated that resuscitation knowledge and skills deteriorate with time and therefore recertification is required for those who have not recently undertaken the course. Recertification provides the opportunity to refresh resuscitation skills and to be updated on resuscitation guidelines, and can be undertaken by attending a provider course or an accredited recertification course. All ALS providers have a responsibility to maintain their skills in resuscitation and to keep up to date with changes in guidelines and practice, and the requirement for recertification should be seen as an absolute minimum frequency of refreshing skills and knowledge.

## Further reading

Nolan JP, Deakin CD, Soar J, Bottiger BW, Smith G. European Resuscitation Council Guidelines for Resuscitation 2005. Section 4: Adult advanced life support. Resuscitation 2005;67 Suppl 1:S39-86.

International Liaison Committee on Resuscitation. 2005 International Consensus on Cardiopulmonary Resuscitation and Emergency Cardiovascular Care Science with Treatment Recommendations. Resuscitation 2005;67:157-341.

Pell JP, Sirel JM, Marsden AK, Ford I, Walker NL, Cobbe SM. Presentation, management, and outcome of out of hospital cardiopulmonary arrest: comparison by underlying aetiology. Heart 2003;89:839-42.

Atwood C, Eisenberg MS, Herlitz J, Rea TD. Incidence of EMS-treated out-of-hospital cardiac arrest in Europe. Resuscitation 2005;67:75-80.

Hodgetts TJ, Kenward G, Vlackonikolis I, et al. Incidence, location and reasons for avoidable in-hospital cardiac arrest in a district general hospital. Resuscitation 2002;54:115-23.

# Adult Advanced Life Support Algorithm

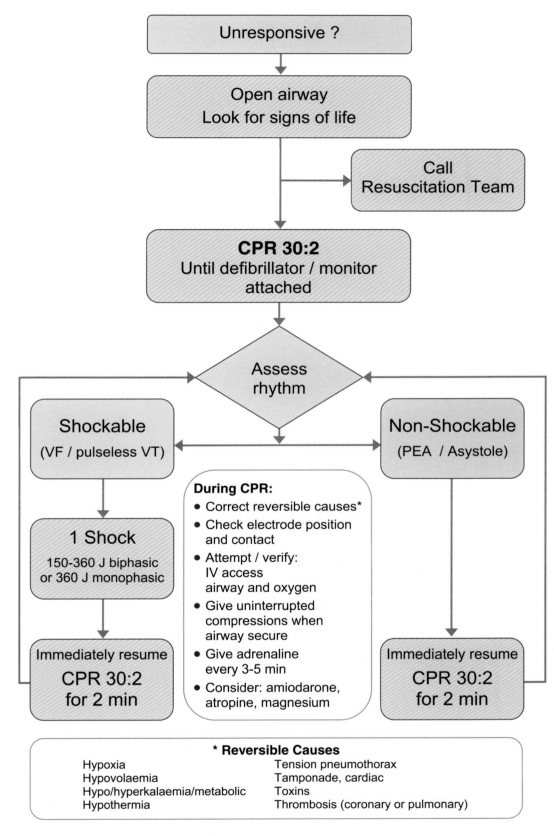

**Figure 1.2  Adult Advanced Life Support Algorithm**

ALS

ALS

# Recognition of the Critically Ill Patient and Prevention of Cardiorespiratory Arrest

## Objectives

To understand:

▶ **The importance of early recognition of the critically ill patient.**

▶ **The causes of cardiorespiratory arrest in adults.**

▶ **How to identify and treat patients at risk of cardiorespiratory arrest using the ABCDE approach.**

## Introduction

Most people who have a cardiorespiratory arrest die. Survivors from in-hospital cardiac arrest usually have a witnessed and monitored VF arrest, primary myocardial ischaemia as the cause, and receive immediate and successful defibrillation.

Most cardiorespiratory arrests in hospital are not sudden or unpredictable events: in approximately 80% of cases there is deterioration in clinical signs during the few hours before cardiac arrest. These patients often have slow and progressive physiological deterioration, often involving hypoxia and hypotension that is unnoticed by staff, or is recognised but treated poorly. The cardiac arrest rhythm in this group is usually non-shockable (PEA or asystole) and the survival rate to hospital discharge is very low.

Early recognition and effective treatment of critically ill patients might prevent some cardiac arrests, deaths and unanticipated intensive care unit (ICU) admissions. Early recognition also helps to identify individuals for whom cardiorespiratory resuscitation is not appropriate or do not wish to be resuscitated.

## Recognising the critically ill patient

In general, the clinical signs of critical illness are similar whatever the underlying process because they reflect failing respiratory, cardiovascular, and neurological systems i.e., ABCDE problems (see below). Abnormal physiology is common on general wards, yet the measurement and recording of important physiological observations of acutely ill patients occurs less frequently than is desirable. The assessment of very simple vital signs, such as respiratory rate, may help to predict cardiorespiratory arrest. To help early detection of critical illness, many hospitals now use early warning scores (EWS) or calling criteria. Early warning scoring systems allocate points to measurements of routine vital signs on the basis of their derangement from an arbitrarily agreed 'normal' range. The weighted score of one or more vital sign observations, or the total EWS, indicates the level of intervention required, e.g., increased frequency of vital signs monitoring, or calling ward doctors or resuscitation teams to the patient. Alternatively, systems incorporating calling criteria are based on routine observations, which activate a response when one or more variables reach an extremely abnormal value. It is not clear which of these two systems is better.

Even when doctors are alerted to a patient's abnormal physiology, there is often delay in attending to the patient or referring to higher levels of care.

## Response to critical illness

The traditional response to cardiac arrest is reactive: the name 'cardiac arrest team' implies that it will be called only after cardiac arrest has occurred. In some hospitals the cardiac arrest team has been replaced by other resuscitation teams. For example, the medical emergency team (MET) responds not only to patients in cardiac arrest, but also to those with acute physiological deterioration. The MET usually comprises medical and nursing staff from intensive care and general medicine and responds to specific calling criteria (Table 2.1). Any member of the healthcare team can initiate a MET call. Early involvement of the MET may reduce cardiac arrests, deaths and unanticipated ICU admissions. MET interventions often involve simple tasks such as starting oxygen therapy and intravenous fluids. The benefits of the MET system remain to be proved.

In the UK, a system of pre-emptive ward care known as critical care outreach, has developed. Outreach services exist in many forms ranging from a single nurse to a 24-hour, seven days per week multiprofessional team. An outreach team or system may reduce ward deaths, postoperative adverse events, ICU admissions and readmissions, and increase survival.

All critically ill patients should be admitted to an area that can provide the greatest supervision and the highest level of organ support and nursing care. This is usually in a critical care area e.g., ICU, high dependency unit (HDU), or resuscitation room. These areas should be staffed by doctors and nurses experienced in advanced resuscitation and critical care skills.

Hospital staffing tends to be at its lowest during the night and at weekends. This influences patient monitoring, treatment and outcomes. Admission to general wards in the evening or to hospital at weekends is associated with increased mortality. Some studies have shown that in-hospital cardiac arrests occurring in the late afternoon or night are more often non-witnessed and have a lower survival rate. Patients discharged at night from ICUs to general wards have an increased risk of in-hospital death compared to those discharged during the day and those discharged to HDUs.

**TABLE 2.1. MEDICAL EMERGENCY TEAM CALLING CRITERIA**

| Acute Change in: | Physiology: |
|---|---|
| Airway | Threatened |
| Breathing | All respiratory arrests<br>Respiratory rate < 5 min$^{-1}$<br>Respiratory rate > 36 min$^{-1}$ |
| Circulation | All cardiac arrests<br>Pulse rate < 40 beats min$^{-1}$<br>Pulse rate > 140 beats min$^{-1}$<br>Systolic blood pressure < 90 mmHg |
| Neurology | Sudden decrease in level of consciousness<br>Decrease in GCS of > 2 points<br>Repeated or prolonged seizures |
| Other | Any patient causing concern who does not fit the above criteria |

# Causes of cardiorespiratory arrest

Cardiorespiratory arrest can be caused by a primary airway, breathing or cardiovascular problem.

## Airway obstruction

For a detailed review of airway management see Chapter 6.

### Causes

Airway obstruction can be complete or partial. Complete airway obstruction will rapidly cause cardiac arrest. Partial obstruction often precedes complete obstruction. Partial airway obstruction may cause cerebral or pulmonary oedema, exhaustion, secondary apnoea, and hypoxic brain injury, and eventually cardiac arrest.

**CAUSES OF AIRWAY OBSTRUCTION**

- Central nervous system depression
- Blood
- Vomitus
- Foreign body (e.g., tooth, food)
- Direct trauma to face or throat
- Epiglottitis
- Pharyngeal swelling (e.g., infection, oedema)
- Laryngospasm
- Bronchospasm
- Bronchial secretions

Central nervous system depression may cause loss of airway patency and protective reflexes. Causes include head injury and intracerebral disease, hypercarbia, the depressant effect of metabolic disorders (e.g., diabetes mellitus), and drugs, including alcohol, opioids and general anaesthetic agents. Laryngospasm can occur with upper airway stimulation in a semi-conscious patient whose airway reflexes remain intact.

### Recognition

Assess the patency of the airway in anyone at risk of obstruction. A conscious patient will complain of difficulty in breathing, may be choking, and will be distressed. With partial airway obstruction, efforts at breathing will be noisy. With complete airway obstruction, respiration will be silent and there will be no air movement at the patient's mouth. Any respiratory movements are usually strenuous. The accessory muscles of respiration will be involved, causing a 'see-saw' or 'rocking-horse' pattern of chest and abdominal movement: the chest is drawn in and the abdomen expands on inspiration, and the opposite occurs on expiration.

### Treatment

The priority is to ensure that the airway remains patent. Treat any problem that places the airway at risk; for example, suck blood and gastric contents from the airway and, unless contraindicated, turn the patient on their side. Give oxygen as soon as possible. Assume actual or impending airway obstruction in anyone with a depressed level of consciousness, regardless of cause. Take steps to safeguard the airway and prevent further complications such as aspiration of gastric contents. This may involve nursing the patient on their side or with a head-up tilt, simple airway opening manoeuvres (head tilt/chin lift or jaw thrust), insertion of an oropharyngeal or nasal airway, elective tracheal intubation or tracheostomy, and insertion of a nasogastric tube to empty the stomach.

## Breathing problems

### Causes

Breathing inadequacy may be acute or chronic. It may be continuous or intermittent, and severe enough to cause apnoea, which will cause a cardiac arrest rapidly. Respiratory arrest often occurs because of a combination of factors; for example, in a patient with chronic respiratory inadequacy, a chest infection, muscle weakness, or fractured ribs may lead to exhaustion, further depressing respiratory function. If breathing is insufficient to oxygenate the blood adequately, a cardiac arrest will occur eventually.

### Respiratory drive

Central nervous system depression may decrease or abolish respiratory drive. The causes are the same as those for airway obstruction from central nervous system depression.

### Respiratory effort

The main respiratory muscles are the diaphragm and intercostal muscles. The latter are innervated at the level of their respective ribs and may be paralysed by a spinal cord lesion above this level. The innervation of the diaphragm is at the level of the third, fourth and fifth segment of the spinal cord. Spontaneous breathing cannot occur with severe cervical cord damage above this level.

Inadequate respiratory effort, caused by muscle weakness or nerve damage, occurs with many diseases (e.g., myasthenia gravis, Guillain-Barré syndrome, and multiple sclerosis). Chronic malnourishment and severe long-term illness may also contribute to generalised weakness.

Breathing may be impaired with restrictive chest wall abnormalities such as kyphoscoliosis. Pain from fractured ribs or sternum will prevent deep breaths and coughing.

### Lung disorders

Lung function is impaired by a pneumothorax or haemothorax. A tension pneumothorax causes a rapid failure of gas exchange, a reduction of venous return to the heart, and a fall in cardiac output. Severe lung disease will impair gas exchange. Causes include infection, aspiration, exacerbation of chronic obstructive pulmonary disease (COPD), asthma, pulmonary embolus, lung contusion, acute respiratory distress syndrome (ARDS) and pulmonary oedema.

## Recognition

A conscious patient will complain of shortness of breath and be distressed. The history and examination will usually indicate the underlying cause. Hypoxia and hypercarbia can cause irritability, confusion, lethargy and a decrease in the level of consciousness. Cyanosis may be visible but is a late sign. A fast respiratory rate (>30 min$^{-1}$) is a useful, simple indicator of breathing problems. Pulse oximetry is an easy, non-invasive measure of the adequacy of oxygenation. However, it is not a reliable indicator of ventilation and an arterial blood gas sample is necessary to obtain values for arterial carbon dioxide tension ($PaCO_2$) and pH. A rising $PaCO_2$ and a decrease in pH are often late signs in a patient with severe respiratory problems.

## Treatment

Give oxygen to all hypoxic patients and treat the underlying cause. For example, suspect a tension pneumothorax from a history of chest trauma and confirm by clinical signs and symptoms. If diagnosed, decompress it immediately by inserting a large bore (14G) cannula into the second intercostal space, in the mid-clavicular line (needle thoracocentesis).

Patients who are having difficulty breathing or are becoming tired will need respiratory support. Non-invasive ventilation using a face mask or a helmet can be useful and prevent the need for tracheal intubation and ventilation. For patients who cannot breathe adequately, sedation, tracheal intubation and controlled ventilation is needed.

## Circulation problems

## Causes

In a few cases of cardiac arrest no causative abnormalities are found. Circulation problems may be caused by primary heart disease or by heart abnormalities secondary to other problems. The heart may stop suddenly or may produce an inadequate cardiac output for a period of time before stopping.

### Primary heart problems

The commonest cause of sudden cardiac arrest is an arrhythmia caused by either ischaemia or myocardial infarction. Cardiac arrest can also be caused by arrhythmia due to other forms of heart disease, by heart block, electrocution and some drugs.

---

**CAUSES OF VENTRICULAR FIBRILLATION**

- Acute coronary syndromes (Chapter 3)
- Hypertensive heart disease
- Valve disease
- Drugs (e.g., antiarrhythmic drugs, tricyclic antidepressants, digoxin)
- Hereditary cardiac diseases e.g., long QT syndromes
- Acidosis
- Abnormal electrolyte concentration (e.g., potassium, magnesium, calcium)
- Hypothermia
- Electrocution

---

Sudden cardiac arrest may also occur with cardiac failure, cardiac tamponade, cardiac rupture, myocarditis and hypertrophic cardiomyopathy.

### Secondary heart problems

The heart is affected by changes elsewhere in the body. For example, cardiac arrest will occur rapidly following asphyxia from airway obstruction or apnoea, tension pneumothorax, or acute severe blood loss. Severe hypoxia and anaemia, hypothermia, oligaemia and severe septic shock will also impair cardiac function and this may lead to cardiac arrest.

## Recognition

The signs and symptoms of cardiac disease include chest pain, shortness of breath, tachycardia, bradycardia, tachypnoea, hypotension, poor peripheral perfusion (prolonged capillary refill time), altered mental state, and oliguria.

Most sudden cardiac deaths occur in people with pre-existing cardiac disease, which may have been unrecognised previously. Although the risk is greater for patients with known severe cardiac disease, most sudden cardiac deaths occur in people with unrecognised disease. Asymptomatic or silent cardiac disease may include hypertensive heart disease, aortic valve disease, cardiomyopathy, myocarditis, and coronary disease.

A few sudden cardiac deaths occur in people without any previous history and with an apparently normal heart. Victims tend to be young, active and otherwise healthy. Risk factors for cardiac disease include increasing age, a strong family history, being male, smoking, diabetes mellitus, hyperlipidaemia and hypertension. An increasing number of cardiac conditions are known to be inherited, including hypertrophic cardiomyopathy, arrhythmogenic right ventricular cardiomyopathy and hereditary long QT syndromes.

ALS

Most successful prevention focuses on treating the underlying cardiac disease. The most common presentation of coronary artery disease is chest pain (Chapter 3).

### Treatment

A comprehensive description of the management of acute coronary syndromes (ACS) is given in Chapter 3. Immediate general treatment for ACS should include:

- Oxygen, in a high concentration.

- Aspirin 300 mg, orally, crushed or chewed, as soon as possible.

- Nitroglycerine, as sublingual glyceryl trinitrate (tablet or spray).

- Morphine (or diamorphine) titrated intravenously to avoid sedation and respiratory depression.

Most patients with cardiac ischaemic pain will be more comfortable sitting up. In some instances lying flat may provoke or worsen the pain. Consider using an anti-emetic, especially if nausea is present.

Survivors of a previous episode of VF are likely to have a further episode unless preventative treatment is given. These patients may need percutaneous coronary intervention, coronary artery bypass grafting, or an implantable defibrillator.

Treating the underlying cause should prevent many secondary cardiac arrests; for example, early goal-directed therapy to optimise vital organ perfusion decreases the risk of death in severe sepsis. Cardiovascular support includes correction of underlying electrolyte or acid-base disturbances, and treatment to achieve a desirable cardiac rate, rhythm and output. Advanced cardiovascular monitoring with a pulmonary artery catheter (or non-invasive system) and echocardiography may be indicated. Appropriate manipulation of cardiac filling may require fluid therapy and vasoactive drugs. Inotropic drugs and vasoconstrictors may be indicated to support cardiac output and blood pressure. In some situations, mechanical circulatory support (e.g., intra-aortic balloon pump) or consideration of heart transplantation will be necessary.

# The ABCDE approach

## Underlying principles

The approach to all critically ill patients is the same. The underlying principles are:

1. Use the **A**irway, **B**reathing, **C**irculation, **D**isability, and **E**xposure approach to assess and treat the patient.

2. Do a complete initial assessment and re-assess regularly.

3. Treat life-threatening problems before moving to the next part of assessment.

4. Assess the effects of treatment.

5. Recognise when you will need extra help. Call for help early.

6. Use all members of the team. This enables interventions, e.g., assessment, attaching monitors, intravenous access, to be undertaken simultaneously.

7. Communicate effectively.

8. The aim of the initial treatment is to keep the patient alive, and achieve some clinical improvement. This will buy time for further treatment.

9. Remember - it can take a few minutes for treatments to work.

## First steps

1. Ensure personal safety.

2. First look at the patient in general to see if the patient appears unwell.

3. If the patient is awake, ask "How are you?" If the patient appears unconscious or has collapsed, shake him and ask "Are you alright?" If he responds normally he has a patent airway, is breathing and has brain perfusion. If he speaks only in short sentences, he may have breathing problems. Failure of the patient to respond is a clear marker of critical illness.

4. Monitor the vital signs early. Attach a pulse oximeter, ECG monitor and a non-invasive blood pressure monitor to all critically ill patients, as soon as possible.

5. Insert an intravenous cannula as soon as possible. Take bloods for investigation when inserting the intravenous cannula.

## Airway (A)

Airway obstruction is an emergency. Get expert help immediately. Untreated, airway obstruction causes hypoxia and risks damage to the brain, kidneys and heart, cardiac arrest, and even death.

1. Look for the signs of airway obstruction:

   - Airway obstruction causes paradoxical chest and abdominal movements ('see-saw' respirations) and the use of the accessory muscles of respiration. Central cyanosis is a late sign of airway obstruction. In complete airway obstruction, there are no breath sounds at the mouth or nose. In partial obstruction, air entry is diminished and often noisy.

   - In the critically ill patient, depressed consciousness often leads to airway obstruction.

2. Treat airway obstruction as a medical emergency:

   - Obtain expert help immediately. Untreated, airway obstruction causes hypoxia (low $PaO_2$) with the risk of hypoxic injury to the brain, kidneys and heart, cardiac arrest, and even death.

**ALS**

- In most cases, only simple methods of airway clearance are required (e.g., airway opening manoeuvres, airways suction, insertion of an oropharyngeal or nasopharyngeal airway). Tracheal intubation may be required when these fail.

3. Give oxygen at high concentration:

- Provide high concentration oxygen using a mask with an oxygen reservoir. Ensure that the oxygen flow is sufficient (usually > 10 l min$^{-1}$) to prevent collapse of the reservoir during inspiration. If the patient's trachea is intubated, give high concentration oxygen with a self-inflating bag.

- In acute respiratory failure, maintain the PaO$_2$ as close to normal as possible (approximately 13 kPa or 100 mmHg). In some patients this is not possible so you may have to tolerate lower values, i.e., at least above 8 kPa (60 mmHg) or 90-92% saturation on a pulse oximeter.

## Breathing (B)

During the immediate assessment of breathing, it is vital to diagnose and treat immediately life-threatening conditions, e.g., acute severe asthma, pulmonary oedema, tension pneumothorax, massive haemothorax.

1. Look, listen and feel for the general signs of respiratory distress: sweating, central cyanosis, use of the accessory muscles of respiration, abdominal breathing.

2. Count the respiratory rate. The normal rate is 12-20 breaths min$^{-1}$. A high, or increasing, respiratory rate is a marker of illness and a warning that the patient may deteriorate suddenly.

3. Assess the depth of each breath, the pattern (rhythm) of respiration and whether chest expansion is equal on both sides.

4. Note any chest deformity (this may increase the risk of deterioration in the ability to breathe normally); look for a raised JVP (e.g., in acute severe asthma or a tension pneumothorax); note the presence and patency of any chest drains; remember that abdominal distension may limit diaphragmatic movement, thereby worsening respiratory distress.

5. Record the inspired oxygen concentration (%) given to the patient and the SpO$_2$ reading of the pulse oximeter (normally 97-100%). The pulse oximeter does not detect hypercapnia. If the patient is receiving supplemental oxygen, the SpO$_2$ may be normal in the presence of a very high PaCO$_2$.

6. Listen to the patient's breath sounds a short distance from his face: rattling airway noises indicate the presence of airway secretions, usually caused by the inability of the patient to cough sufficiently or to take a deep breath. Stridor or wheeze suggests partial, but significant, airway obstruction.

7. Percuss the chest: hyper-resonance may suggest a

pneumothorax; dullness usually indicates consolidation or pleural fluid.

8. Auscultate the chest: bronchial breathing indicates lung consolidation with patent airways; absent or reduced sounds suggest a pneumothorax or pleural fluid or lung consolidation caused by complete bronchial obstruction.

9. Check the position of the trachea in the suprasternal notch: deviation to one side indicates mediastinal shift (e.g., pneumothorax, lung fibrosis or pleural fluid).

10. Feel the chest wall to detect surgical emphysema or crepitus (suggesting a pneumothorax until proven otherwise).

11. The specific treatment of respiratory disorders depends upon the cause. Nevertheless, all critically ill patients should be given oxygen. In a subgroup of patients with chronic obstructive pulmonary disease (COPD), high concentrations of oxygen may depress breathing. Nevertheless, these patients will also sustain end-organ damage or cardiac arrest if their blood oxygen tensions are allowed to decrease. In this group, aim for a lower than normal PaO$_2$ and oxygen saturation. A suitable target is a PaO$_2$ of 8 kPa (60 mmHg) or 90-92% saturation (SpO$_2$) on pulse oximetry.

12. If the patient's depth or rate of breathing is judged to be inadequate, or absent, use bag-mask or pocket mask ventilation to improve oxygenation and ventilation, whilst calling immediately for expert help.

## Circulation (C)

In almost all medical and surgical emergencies, consider hypovolaemia to be the primary cause of shock, until proven otherwise. Unless there are obvious signs of a cardiac cause, give intravenous fluid to any patient with cool peripheries and a fast heart rate. In surgical patients, rapidly exclude haemorrhage (overt or hidden). Remember that breathing problems, such as a tension pneumothorax, can also compromise a patient's circulatory state. This should have been treated earlier on in the assessment.

1. Look at the colour of the hands and digits: are they blue, pink, pale or mottled?

2. Assess the limb temperature by feeling the patient's hands: are they cool or warm?

3. Measure the capillary refill time (CRT). Apply cutaneous pressure for five seconds on a fingertip held at heart level (or just above) with enough pressure to cause blanching. Time how long it takes for the skin to return to the colour of the surrounding skin after releasing the pressure. The normal value for CRT is usually less than two seconds. A prolonged CRT suggests poor peripheral perfusion. Other factors (e.g., cold surroundings, poor lighting, old age) can prolong CRT.

4. Assess the state of the veins: they may be under-filled or collapsed when hypovolaemia is present.

**ALS**

5.  Count the patient's pulse rate (or preferably heart rate).

6.  Palpate peripheral and central pulses, assessing for presence, rate, quality, regularity and equality. Barely palpable central pulses suggests a poor cardiac output, whilst a bounding pulse may indicate sepsis.

7.  Measure the patient's blood pressure. Even in shock, the blood pressure may be normal, because compensatory mechanisms increase peripheral resistance in response to reduced cardiac output. A low diastolic blood pressure suggests arterial vasodilation (as in anaphylaxis or sepsis). A narrowed pulse pressure (difference between systolic and diastolic pressures; normally ~ 35-45 mmHg) suggests arterial vasoconstriction (cardiogenic shock or hypovolaemia) and may occur with rapid tachyarrhythmia.

8.  Auscultate the heart. Is there a murmur or pericardial rub? Are the heart sounds difficult to hear? Does the audible heart rate correspond to the pulse rate?

9.  Look for other signs of a poor cardiac output, such as reduced conscious level and, if the patient has a urinary catheter, oliguria (urine volume < 0.5 ml kg$^{-1}$ hour$^{-1}$).

10. Look thoroughly for external haemorrhage from wounds or drains or evidence of concealed haemorrhage (e.g., thoracic, intra-peritoneal, retroperitoneal or into gut). Intra-thoracic, intra-abdominal or pelvic blood loss may be significant, even if drains are empty.

11. The specific treatment of cardiovascular collapse depends on the cause, but should be directed at fluid replacement, haemorrhage control and restoration of tissue perfusion. Seek the signs of conditions that are immediately life threatening, e.g., cardiac tamponade, massive or continuing haemorrhage, septicaemic shock, and treat them urgently.

12. Insert one or more large (14 or 16 G) intravenous cannulae. Use short, wide-bore cannulae, because they enable the highest flow.

13. Take blood from the cannula for routine haematological, biochemical, coagulation and microbiological investigations, and cross-matching, before infusing intravenous fluid.

14. Give a rapid fluid challenge (over 5-10 min) of 500 ml of warmed crystalloid solution if the patient is normotensive. Give one litre, if the patient is hypotensive. Use smaller volumes (e.g., 250 ml) for patients with known cardiac failure and use closer monitoring (listen to the chest for crackles after each bolus, consider a CVP line).

15. Reassess the heart rate and BP regularly (every 5 min), aiming for the patient's normal BP or, if this is unknown, a target > 100 mmHg systolic.

16. If the patient does not improve, repeat the fluid challenge.

17. If symptoms and signs of cardiac failure (dyspnoea, increased heart rate, raised JVP, a third heart sound and pulmonary crackles on auscultation) occur, decrease the fluid infusion rate or stop the fluids altogether. Seek alternative means of improving tissue perfusion (e.g. inotropes or vasopressors).

18. If the patient has primary chest pain and a suspected ACS record a 12-lead ECG early, and treat initially with oxygen, aspirin, nitroglycerine, and morphine.

## Disability (D)

Common causes of unconsciousness include profound hypoxia, hypercapnia, cerebral hypoperfusion, or the recent administration of sedatives or analgesic drugs.

1.  Review and treat the ABCs: exclude or treat hypoxia and hypotension.

2.  Check the patient's drug chart for reversible drug-induced causes of depressed consciousness. Give an antagonist where appropriate (e.g., naloxone for opioid toxicity).

3.  Examine the pupils (size, equality and reaction to light).

4.  Make a rapid initial assessment of the patient's conscious level using the AVPU method: **A**lert, responds to **V**ocal stimuli, responds to **P**ainful stimuli or **U**nresponsive to all stimuli. Alternatively use the Glasgow Coma Scale score.

5.  Measure the blood glucose using a glucose meter or stick method to exclude hypoglycaemia. If below 3 mmol l$^{-1}$, give 50 ml of 10% glucose solution intravenously.

6.  Nurse unconscious patients in the lateral position if their airway is not protected.

## Exposure (E)

To examine the patient properly full exposure of the body may be necessary. Respect the patient's dignity and minimise heat loss.

## Additional information

1.  Take a full clinical history from the patient, his relatives or friends, and other staff.

2.  Review the patient's notes and charts:
    a.  Study both absolute and trended values of vital signs.
    b.  Check that important routine medications are prescribed and being given.

3.  Review the results of laboratory or radiological investigations.

4.  Consider which level of care is required by the patient (e.g., ward, HDU, ICU).

5.  Make complete entries in the patient's notes of your findings, assessment and treatment. Record the patient's response to therapy.

6.  Consider definitive treatment of the patient's underlying condition.

## Key learning points

- Most patients who have an in-hospital cardiac arrest have warning signs and symptoms before the arrest.

- Early recognition and treatment of critically ill patients will prevent some cardiorespiratory arrests.

- Use strategies such as early warning scoring systems to identify patients at risk of cardiorespiratory arrest.

- Airway, breathing and circulation problems can cause cardiorespiratory arrest.

- Use the ABCDE approach to assess and treat critically ill patients.

## Further reading

International Liaison Committee on Resuscitation. Part 4. Advanced Life Support 2005 International Consensus on Cardiopulmonary Resuscitation and Emergency Cardiovascular Care Science with Treatment Recommendations. Resuscitation 2005;67:213-247.

Nolan JP, Deakin CD, Soar J, Bottiger BW, Smith G. European Resuscitation Council Guidelines for Resuscitation 2005. Section 4: Adult advanced life support. Resuscitation 2005;Suppl 1:S39-86.

National Confidential Enquiry into Patient Outcome and Death. An Acute Problem? London: National Confidential Enquiry into Patient Outcome and Death; 2005.

Cretikos M, Parr M, Hillman K, et al. Guidelines for the uniform reporting of data for medical emergency teams. Resuscitation 2006;68:11-25.

Smith GB, Osgood VM, Crane S. ALERT - a multiprofessional training course in the care of the acutely ill adult patient. Resuscitation 2002;52:281-286.

ALS

ALS

# Acute Coronary Syndromes

## Objectives

To understand:

▶ **The disease process which gives rise to acute coronary syndromes.**

▶ **How to differentiate between the acute coronary syndromes.**

▶ **The immediate treatment of acute coronary syndromes.**

▶ **Management of patients after recovery from an acute coronary syndrome.**

## Introduction

Whilst rapid resuscitation offers the best chance of recovery from cardiac arrest, it is clearly better to prevent cardiac arrest whenever possible. Many cardiac arrests are caused by underlying coronary artery disease and occur in the context of an acute coronary syndrome (ACS). It is therefore important that the ALS provider understands how to recognise an ACS, how to assess a patient with an ACS, and what treatments may reduce the risk of cardiac arrest and death.

## Definitions and pathogenesis

The acute coronary syndromes (ACS) comprise:

- Unstable angina

- Non-ST segment elevation myocardial infarction

- ST segment elevation myocardial infarction

These clinical syndromes form parts of a spectrum of the same disease process. In the vast majority of cases this process is initiated by the fissuring of an atheromatous plaque in a coronary artery causing:

- haemorrhage into the plaque causing it to swell and restrict the lumen of the artery;

- contraction of smooth muscle within the artery wall, causing further constriction of the lumen;

- thrombus formation on the surface of the plaque, which may cause partial or complete obstruction of the lumen of the artery, or distal embolism.

The extent to which these events reduce the flow of blood to the myocardium largely determines the nature of the clinical ACS that ensues.

## Angina (stable and unstable)

Angina is pain or discomfort caused by myocardial ischaemia and is felt usually in or across the centre of the chest as tightness or an indigestion-like ache. As with acute myocardial infarction (AMI), the pain/discomfort often radiates into the throat, into one or both arms (more commonly the left), and into the back or into the epigastrium. Some patients experience angina predominantly in one or more of these areas rather than in the chest. Many patients perceive it as discomfort rather than pain. As with AMI, angina is sometimes accompanied by belching and this may be misinterpreted as evidence of indigestion as the cause of the discomfort. Pain of this nature, which is provoked only by exercise and which settles promptly when exercise ceases, is referred to as stable angina and is not an ACS.

In contrast, **unstable angina** is defined by one or more of:

1. Angina of effort occurring over a few days with increasing frequency provoked by progressively less exertion. This is referred to as 'crescendo angina'.

2. Episodes of angina occurring recurrently and unpredictably, without specific provocation by exercise. These episodes may be relatively short-lived (e.g., a few minutes) and may settle spontaneously or be relieved temporarily by sublingual glyceryl trinitrate, before recurring within a few hours.

3. An unprovoked and prolonged episode of chest pain, raising suspicion of AMI, but without definite ECG or laboratory evidence of AMI (see below).

In unstable angina, the ECG may:
a) be normal;
b) show evidence of acute myocardial ischaemia (usually ST segment depression);
c) show non-specific abnormalities (e.g., T wave inversion).

In unstable angina, cardiac enzymes are usually normal (but remember that there are causes other than myocardial infarction for elevated muscle enzymes such as CK), and troponin release is absent or very minor. ECG abnormality, especially ST segment depression, is a marker of increased risk of further coronary events in patients with unstable angina. Troponin release is also a marker of increased risk and risk increases with the level of troponin. However, a normal ECG and absent troponin release does not necessarily mean that a patient with unstable angina is not at high risk of early further life-threatening coronary events. Only if the ECG and other markers of coronary risk (e.g., troponin) are normal, and further risk assessment (e.g., by exercise testing) does not indicate evidence of reversible myocardial ischaemia, should other possible causes of acute chest pain be considered if the initial history suggested unstable angina.

## Non-ST segment elevation myocardial infarction (NSTEMI)

Acute myocardial infarction typically presents with chest pain that is felt as a heaviness or tightness or indigestion-like discomfort in the chest or upper abdomen, usually sustained for at least 20-30 min, often longer. The chest pain/discomfort often radiates into the throat, into one or both arms (more commonly the left), into the back or into the epigastrium. Some patients experience the discomfort predominantly in one or more of these other areas rather than in the chest. Sometimes it may be accompanied by belching and this may be misinterpreted as evidence of indigestion as the cause of the discomfort.

Some patients present with chest pain suggestive of AMI and non-specific ECG abnormalities such as ST segment depression or T wave inversion (Figures 3.1, 3.2). In a patient with a history suggestive of ACS and laboratory tests showing substantial release of troponin (with or without elevated plasma concentrations of cardiac enzymes) this indicates that myocardial damage has occurred. This is referred to as NSTEMI. In this situation it is less likely that there has been abrupt complete occlusion of the culprit artery than in ST segment elevation MI (STEMI).

The amount of troponin or cardiac enzyme released reflects the extent of myocardial damage. Some of these patients will be at high risk of progression to coronary occlusion, more extensive myocardial damage, and sudden arrhythmic death. The risk of this is highest in the first few hours, days and months after the index event and diminishes progressively with time.

NSTEMI and unstable angina are classified together as 'non ST segment elevation ACS' because the treatment of the two is essentially the same and differs in some respects from the treatment of STEMI. Treatment is dictated largely by assessment of risk.

## ST segment elevation myocardial infarction (STEMI)

A history of sustained acute chest pain typical of AMI, accompanied by acute ST segment elevation on a 12-lead ECG is the basis for diagnosis of STEMI.

These findings almost always indicate on-going myocardial damage caused by acute complete occlusion of the 'culprit' coronary artery (after initial plaque fissuring). Left untreated there is likely to be further myocardial damage in the territory of the occluded artery, usually reflected in the development of Q waves on the ECG. During the acute phase of STEMI there is a substantial risk of ventricular tachycardia (VT) and ventricular fibrillation (VF) and sudden death (Figure 3.3).

# Diagnosis of acute coronary syndromes

## History

An accurate history is a crucial first step in establishing a diagnosis, but there are potential sources of confusion. Some patients (e.g., the elderly, diabetics, during the peri-operative period) may develop an ACS with little or no chest discomfort. The pain of angina or myocardial infarction is often mistaken for indigestion both by patients and healthcare professionals. Symptoms such as belching, nausea or vomiting are not helpful in distinguishing cardiac

pain from indigestion; all may accompany angina and myocardial infarction.

## Clinical examination

Clinical examination is of limited benefit in the diagnosis of ACS. Severe pain of any source may provoke some of the clinical signs, such as sweating, pallor and tachycardia, which commonly accompany ACS. Examination may identify an alternative, obvious cause for chest pain (e.g., localised severe chest wall tenderness).

Examination may identify other important abnormalities (e.g., a cardiac murmur or signs of heart failure) that will influence choices of investigation and treatment. In patients with acute chest pain remember also to check for evidence of aortic dissection, especially if thrombolytic therapy is intended. The presence of aortic dissection may be suggested by clinical signs such as loss of a pulse or asymmetry of the pulses in the upper limbs, acute aortic regurgitation, or signs of stroke from carotid artery involvement. Suspect aortic dissection in any patient whose acute chest pain is accompanied by marked hypotension but no obvious ECG evidence of AMI. However, in a patient with a good history and typical ECG evidence of STEMI do not delay reperfusion therapy without strong clinical evidence to justify prior investigation of possible aortic dissection.

Initial examination also serves as an important baseline so that changes, due either to progression of the underlying condition or in response to treatment, may be detected.

Also suspect extensive right ventricular (RV) infarction in patients with inferior or posterior STEMI who have elevated jugular venous pressure but no evidence of pulmonary oedema. Kussmaul's sign may be positive (JVP increases on inspiration). These patients are often hypotensive.

## Investigations

### The 12-lead ECG

Record a 12-lead ECG as soon as possible during the initial assessment and subsequently to assess progression of the ACS and the response to treatment. The presence of ECG abnormalities on the initial recording may support the clinical suspicion of ACS and indicate the appropriate treatment.

The ECG is a crucial component of risk assessment and planning of treatment. Acute ST segment elevation or new left bundle branch block in a patient with a typical history of AMI is an indication for treatment to try to re-open an occluded coronary artery (reperfusion therapy), either by emergency percutaneous coronary intervention (PCI) or with thrombolytic therapy. In contrast, ST segment depression suggests a low probability of benefit from thrombolytic therapy, regardless of whether the ultimate diagnostic label is unstable angina or NSTEMI. In unstable angina, the presence of ST segment depression indicates a higher risk of further coronary events than if ST segment depression is absent. These higher risk patients require immediate medical treatment (e.g., low-molecular-weight heparin, aspirin, clopidogrel, beta blockade, glycoprotein IIb/IIIa inhibitor),

ALS

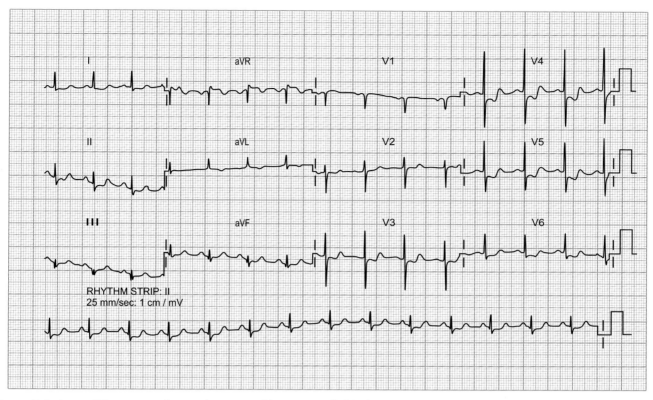

**Figure 3.1  Acute ST segment depression caused by myocardial ischaemia in a patient with a non-ST segment elevation ACS**

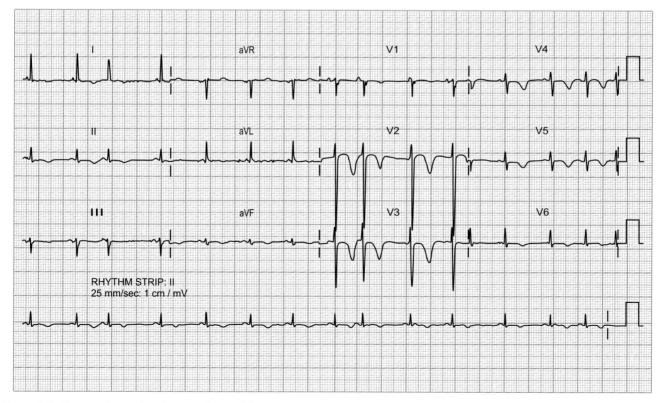

**Figure 3.2  T wave inversion in a patient with NSTEMI**

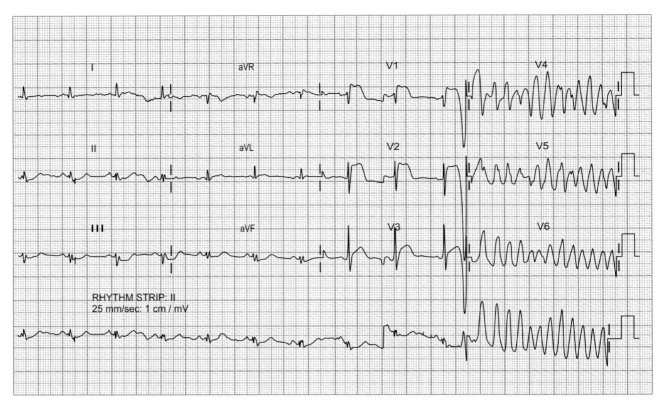

**Figure 3.3  Onset of VF during an ECG recording in a patient with an acute anteroseptal STEMI**

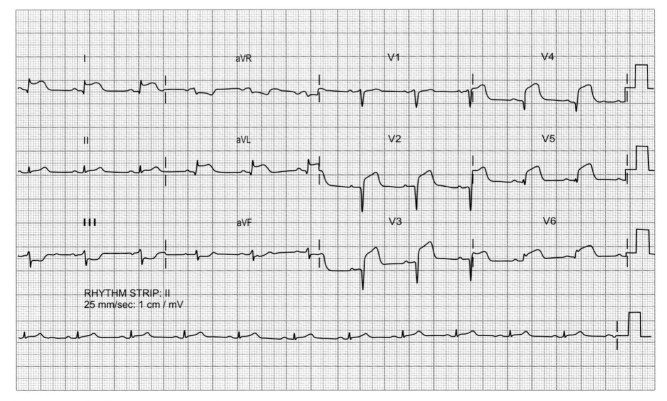

**Figure 3.4  12-lead ECG - Anteroseptal STEMI**

ALS

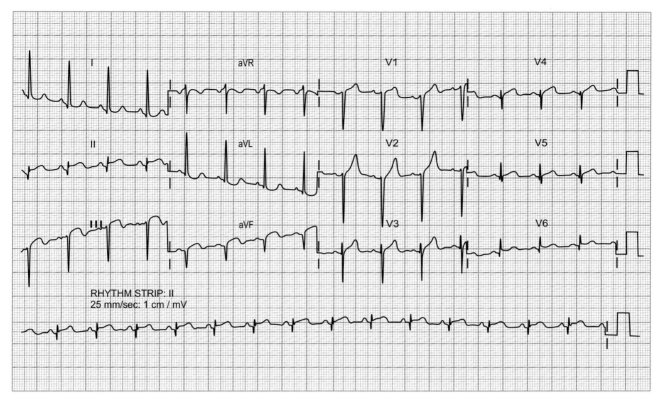

**Figure 3.5  12-lead ECG – Inferior STEMI**

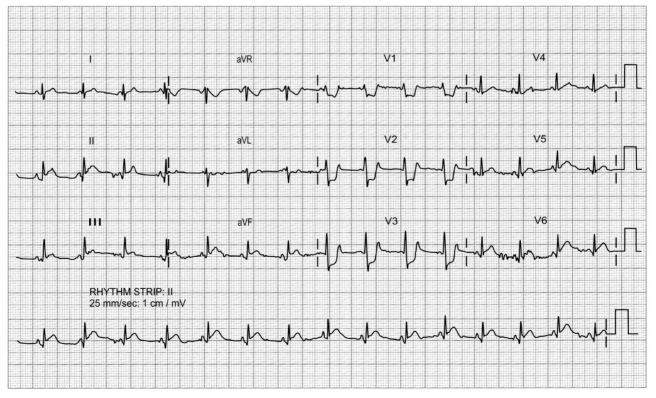

**Figure 3.6  12-lead ECG – Posterior STEMI**

Original kindly supplied by Dean Jenkins

prompt investigation by coronary angiography, and often revascularisation by PCI, or coronary artery bypass surgery.

The ECG provides some information about the site and extent of myocardial damage in AMI particularly in STEMI. This is important since the site and extent of myocardial ischaemia or damage influences prognosis and, in some cases, the appropriate choice of treatment:

1. Anterior or anteroseptal infarction (Figure 3.4) is seen usually in leads V1-V4 and is almost always caused by a lesion in the left anterior descending (LAD) coronary artery. An anterior MI has a worse prognosis and is more likely to cause impairment of left ventricular function. These patients therefore benefit more from immediate reperfusion therapy and early treatment with an angiotensin converting enzyme inhibitor (ACEI).

2. Inferior infarction is seen usually in leads II, III, and aVF (Figure 3.5), and is caused often by a lesion in the right coronary artery or, less commonly, the circumflex artery.

3. Lateral infarction is seen usually in leads V5-V6 and/or leads I and aVL (sometimes aVL alone) and is caused often by a lesion in the circumflex artery or diagonal branch of the LAD artery.

4. Posterior myocardial infarction is usually recognised when there is a reciprocal change in the anterior chest leads (Figure 3.6). ST segment depression in these leads reflects posterior ST elevation, and development of a dominant R wave reflects posterior Q wave development. This is also most commonly due to a right coronary artery lesion but may be caused by a circumflex artery lesion in those people in whom this artery provides the main blood supply to the posterior part of the left ventricle and septum. Suspicion of a posterior infarction can be confirmed by repeating the ECG with posterior leads. These leads (V8, V9 and V10) are placed in a horizontal line around the chest, continuing from V6 (mid-axillary line) and V7 (posterior axillary line). V9 is placed to the left of the spine, V8 half way between V7 and V9 and V10 to the right of the spine.

Right ventricular (RV) infarction may be present in up to one third of patients with inferior and posterior STEMI. Extensive RV infarction may be seen on a conventional 12-lead ECG when ST segment elevation in lead V1 accompanies an inferior or posterior STEMI; use of right-sided precordial leads, especially V4R can also be useful in detecting RV infarction. In this case right-sided precordial leads, particularly V4R, may reveal RV infarction. Two-dimensional echocardiography is also very useful. A diagnosis of extensive RV infarction is suggested by fluid-responsive hypotension and signs of high CVP (as jugular venous distension) without pulmonary congestion. In these patients nitrates should be avoided.

The ST segment depression and T wave inversion that may occur in NSTEMI are less clearly related to the site of myocardial damage than the changes in STEMI. Remember also that use of modified limb leads for ECG recording may alter the morphology of the 12-lead ECG and in particular the modified inferior leads may not show true electrical activity from the inferior wall of the left ventricle.

## Laboratory tests

The other important components of diagnosis and risk assessment are laboratory tests.

### Cardiac troponins (troponin T and troponin I)

Cardiac-specific troponins are components of the contractile structure of myocardial cells. Because concentrations of troponin in the blood of healthy individuals are undetectably low, and cardiac-specific troponins measured by current assays do not arise from extra-cardiac sources, the troponins are very sensitive and specific markers of cardiac injury. The main value of troponin measurement is in the assessment of risk. In the context of unstable angina, an elevated troponin level 6-8 hours after the onset of pain indicates a higher risk of further coronary events than if the troponin level is normal (i.e., undetectable). A combination of ST segment depression on the ECG and raised troponin identifies a particularly high-risk group for subsequent MI and sudden cardiac death.

The release of troponin does not in itself indicate a diagnosis of ACS. Troponin release is a marker of risk and should be regarded as evidence of NSTEMI only when the history indicates a high probability of AMI. Troponin may be released in many other conditions including myocarditis, acute or chronic heart failure, sustained tachyarrhythmia, pulmonary embolism, renal failure and acute sepsis. As with all clinical evidence, it is essential that troponin results are interpreted in the context of the clinical history.

There is continuing debate over what level of troponin release is regarded (in appropriate clinical and ECG context) as definite evidence of acute myocardial infarction and whether modest troponin release may be regarded in some circumstances as evidence of 'unstable angina with minimal myocardial necrosis', rather than of myocardial infarction. Further clarification of this issue is likely to emerge at national and international levels. Furthermore the appropriate treatment of ACS is a rapidly evolving field, as new evidence and new treatments emerge. ALS providers are encouraged to maintain up-to-date awareness of new therapeutic developments and of new agreed definitions that will guide the appropriate assessment and treatment of patients with acute coronary syndromes.

### Creatine kinase (CK), aspartate transaminase (AST) and lactate dehydrogenase (LDH)

These enzymes are released from cardiac muscle when it is damaged; however, they are released also from skeletal muscle when it is damaged or during prolonged, vigorous exercise. To help clarify whether elevated CK concentrations in the blood originate from cardiac or skeletal muscle, the specific iso-enzyme of CK in cardiac muscle (CK-MB) can be measured. In many hospitals, measurement of CK-MB is not available routinely.

Nevertheless, the amount of CK release from myocardium (e.g., when measured on sequential blood samples over three days) can serve as an approximate measure of the amount of myocardial damage.

### Echocardiography

This can be useful in assessing the severity of LV impairment resulting from any AMI. It is particularly important and urgent in confirming RV dilatation and impairment when extensive RV infarction is suspected, and in identifying some complications of AMI, including acquired ventricular septal defect and severe mitral regurgitation, both of which may require urgent surgical correction.

## Risk assessment

The choice of treatment is determined largely by the risk of immediate extensive myocardial damage or early further coronary events. Accurate risk assessment in ACS enables early treatment to reduce risk and thereby prevent some instances of cardiac arrest and sudden death.

## Immediate treatment

## General measures in all acute coronary syndromes

Start with rapid clinical assessment and ECG. Give immediate treatment to relieve symptoms, limit myocardial damage and reduce the risk of cardiac arrest. Immediate general treatment for ACS comprises:

- oxygen, in a high concentration;

- aspirin 300 mg, orally, crushed or chewed, as soon as possible;

- nitroglycerine, as sublingual glyceryl trinitrate (tablet or spray) unless patient is hypotensive or extensive RV infarction is suspected;

- morphine (or diamorphine) titrated intravenously to avoid sedation and respiratory depression.

Most patients with cardiac ischaemic pain will be more comfortable sitting up. In some instances lying flat may provoke or worsen the pain. Consider using an anti-emetic, especially if nausea is present.

## Treatment of STEMI (or MI with new left bundle branch block)

Aim to achieve reperfusion therapy without delay - the aim is to restore the blood supply to myocardium that has not yet been damaged irreversibly. Clinical trials have confirmed the effectiveness of reperfusion therapy in reducing infarct size, complications, and mortality from MI.

The risk-benefit ratio for reperfusion therapy favours reperfusion therapy for those patients who are at highest risk of immediate major myocardial damage and death. Reperfusion therapy is most effective when undertaken early after the onset of myocardial infarction and the benefit diminishes progressively with delay. Twelve hours after the onset of the chest pain of AMI, the risks of reperfusion therapy outweigh any small residual benefit, since most myocardial damage caused by coronary artery occlusion will have occurred by this time. This emphasises the importance of early and accurate assessment of patients with MI. However, thrombolytic therapy will not re-open the culprit coronary artery in all patients and this treatment carries some risk of bleeding, including cerebral haemorrhage. The need to achieve reperfusion as early as possible remains a high priority and for those patients for whom primary PCI is not immediately available initial treatment by thrombolytic therapy may offer the best chance of achieving early reperfusion.

### Coronary reperfusion therapy

Coronary reperfusion may be achieved in one of two ways:

- Percutaneous coronary intervention (PCI) may be used to re-open the occluded artery. This is referred to as primary PCI.

- Thrombolytic therapy may be given in an attempt to dissolve the occluding thrombus that precipitated the MI.

In theory, coronary artery bypass surgery (CABG) could be used to restore blood flow beyond the site of occlusion, but in practice this cannot be achieved quickly enough to salvage myocardium and the risk of surgery in this setting is high.

The most important aspect of reperfusion therapy is that reperfusion should be achieved as early as possible after the onset of chest pain. The risk of treatment changes very little if at all with time, but the benefit diminishes rapidly and the maximum benefit is seen when reperfusion therapy is delivered within 1 h of the onset of chest pain.

### Percutaneous coronary intervention (PCI)

The recommended method for reperfusion therapy in STEMI is primary PCI, provided this can be achieved within 90 min of first medical contact. Coronary angiography is used to identify the occluded coronary artery, following which a guidewire is passed through the occluding thrombus, enabling a deflated balloon to be positioned at the site of occlusion and inflated to re-open the artery. It is usual practice to insert a stent into the segment of previously occluded artery, to reduce the risk of restenosis at this point.

The advantages of PCI are:

- reliable re-opening of the culprit artery in the majority of patients;

- visual evidence that the occluded artery has not only been re-opened, but also re-opened to a normal calibre;

- lower risk of major bleeding than with thrombolytic therapy.

Whilst primary PCI is being made more widely available to provide reliable reperfusion therapy, its major limitation is that it requires 24-h availability of a staffed catheter laboratory and an operator skilled in the technique — resources that are not available universally. Where there is

ALS

## Table 3.1 Typical indications for thrombolytic therapy for AMI

Presentation within 12 h of onset of chest pain suggestive of AMI and:

- ST segment elevation > 0·2 mV in 2 adjacent chest leads, or > 0·1 mV in 2 or more 'adjacent' limb leads; or
- Dominant R waves and ST depression in V1-V3 (posterior infarction); or
- New-onset (or presumed new-onset) left bundle branch block.

## Table 3.2 Typical contraindications to thrombolytic therapy

**Absolute**

- Previous haemorrhagic stroke.
- Ischaemic stroke during the previous 6 months.
- Central nervous system damage or neoplasm.
- Recent (within 3 weeks) major surgery, head injury or other major trauma.
- Active internal bleeding (menses excluded) or gastro-intestinal bleeding within the past month.
- Known or suspected aortic dissection.
- Known bleeding disorder.

**Relative**

- Refractory hypertension (systolic blood pressure >180 mmHg).
- Transient ischaemic attack in preceding 6 months.
- Oral anticoagulant treatment.
- Pregnancy or less than 1 week post-partum.
- Traumatic CPR.
- Non-compressible vascular puncture.
- Active peptic ulcer disease.
- Advanced liver disease.
- Infective endocarditis.
- Previous allergic reaction to the thrombolytic drug to be used.

  If streptokinase has been given more than four days previously, use a different thrombolytic agent (antibodies reduce effectiveness).

## Table 3.3 Thrombolytic drugs

**Streptokinase**

- Often causes hypotension and bradycardia, delaying treatment.
- May cause allergy or anaphylaxis.
- Takes at least 1 h (intravenous infusion) to complete.
- Not suitable for pre-hospital therapy.
- Avoid if used previously more than four days beforehand.
- Dose – 1.5 million units in 100 ml 0.9% saline.
- Relatively inexpensive.

**Alteplase (R-tPA)**

- Complex intravenous infusion regimen.
- Slightly more likely to achieve thrombolysis than streptokinase.
- Short-acting – therefore requires heparin for 48 h after administration.
- Dose: 15 mg intravenous bolus, then infusion of 0.75 mg kg$^{-1}$ over 1 h (accelerated regimen).

**Reteplase**

- Similar efficacy to alteplase.
- Simple double-bolus regimen.
- Short-acting – requires heparin for 48 h.
- Dose: intravenous bolus of 10 units, then further intravenous bolus of 10 units after 30 min.

**Tenecteplase**

- Similar efficacy to alteplase.
- Single bolus weight-related dose.
- Short-acting – requires heparin for 48 h.
- Dose: 30-50 mg (6000-10000 units) according to patient weight.

any likelihood of substantial delay in arranging primary angioplasty, thrombolytic therapy may offer the patient the best chance of achieving early reperfusion, and maximum risk reduction.

Evidence is still being accumulated to determine the role of 'facilitated PCI', in which PCI is carried out after initial thrombolytic therapy and the effectiveness of 'rescue PCI' in which PCI is carried out when it is suspected that thrombolytic therapy has failed to re-open the culprit artery, or when there is evidence of re-occlusion after initially successful thrombolytic therapy.

## Thrombolytic therapy

Thrombolytic therapy has been shown in large-scale clinical trials to provide substantial reduction in mortality from AMI when given during the first few hours after the onset of chest pain. One of the major advantages of thrombolytic therapy is that it does not require a cardiac catheter laboratory or an operator skilled in angioplasty. Pre-hospital thrombolytic therapy may achieve early treatment and resulting clinical benefit when transport times to hospital are long (e.g., > 30 min). Earlier treatment may also be achieved by minimising door-to-needle time (time from arrival at hospital to administration of thrombolytic therapy). This may be achieved by giving thrombolytic therapy in the emergency department.

Disadvantages of thrombolytic therapy include its inability to achieve reperfusion in all cases, the limited ability to detect when reperfusion has occurred, and the risk of inducing bleeding.

Table 3.1 lists typical indications for thrombolytic therapy and typical contraindications are shown in Table 3.2. Most of these contra-indications are relative; the experienced clinician will decide whether the benefit from thrombolytic therapy outweighs the risk to the individual patient. Some of the available thrombolytic drugs are listed in Table 3.3.

## Treatment of unstable angina and NSTEMI

The immediate treatment objectives in these syndromes are:

- To prevent new thrombus formation, which may occlude an artery and lead to, or extend, myocardial damage.

- To reduce myocardial oxygen demand, providing myocardial cells with a better chance of survival in the presence of a limited supply of oxygen and glucose.

### Prevention of further thrombus formation

- Give subcutaneous low molecular weight heparin in therapeutic doses (weight-related).

- Start clopidogrel (loading dose at least 300 mg but consider 600 mg or 900 mg if very rapid loading is needed).

- In high risk patients, especially if early PCI is planned, start glycoprotein IIb/IIIa inhibitor (e.g., tirofiban).

### Reduction in oxygen demand

- Start beta-adrenoceptor blockade (unless contra-indicated).

- Consider diltiazem if beta-blockade contra-indicated.

- Avoid dihydropyridine calcium channel blockers (e.g., nifedipine).

- Consider intravenous or buccal nitrate if angina persists or recurs after sublingual nitrate.

- Consider early introduction of an ACEI, especially if there is left ventricular systolic impairment or heart failure.

- Treat complications such as heart failure or tachyarrhythmia promptly and effectively.

# Subsequent management of patients with acute coronary syndromes

## Suspected unstable angina – low risk patients

Patients with suspected unstable angina without a definite history of preceding angina of effort or myocardial infarction and without high-risk features at presentation (ECG and troponin levels normal after 6-8 h) are suitable for early further risk assessment (e.g., by exercise testing).

## Suspected angina – high risk unstable angina and NSTEMI

Patients with unstable angina and high-risk features (resting ST segment depression, positive troponin or early positive exercise test) should be considered for further investigation by coronary angiography during the same hospital admission. Many of these will benefit from revascularisation by PCI. A few may require CABG. Patients with NSTEMI should be regarded similarly as a high-risk group, requiring early assessment by coronary angiography during the same hospital admission in the majority of cases.

## STEMI

In patients with completed STEMI who have not been treated with reperfusion therapy (e.g., because of late presentation), risk stratification by exercise testing may be helpful once the immediate evidence of acute myocardial necrosis (e.g., fever, arrhythmia) has settled and any complications (e.g., heart failure) have been treated effectively.

If thrombolytic therapy has been used, some patients may be left with a severe stenosis or unstable plaque in the culprit coronary artery, and PCI can stabilise this situation and reduce the risk of re-occlusion of the artery, and resulting risk of further myocardial infarction, cardiac arrest and sudden death. Exercise testing may draw attention to such risk but is not highly sensitive or specific in this setting and there is an increasing tendency to include coronary angiography as part of risk assessment before hospital discharge in this group of patients. The role of 'facilitated PCI' (in which initial thrombolytic therapy is followed by

ALS

early coronary angiography and PCI) remains a subject of debate and on-going study.

In patients with suspected extensive RV infarction at presentation, particularly when hypotension is present, avoid the use of nitrates. Intravenous fluid (0.9% saline or colloid) may be needed to increase blood pressure and cardiac output.

## Ventricular arrhythmia complicating acute coronary syndromes

When ventricular arrhythmia complicates an acute coronary syndrome, interpret its significance in the context of the precise clinical setting and the time of onset of the arrhythmia. When VF/VT cardiac arrest occurs within the first 24-48 h after STEMI, and subsequent recovery is uncomplicated, the risk of another ventricular arrhythmia is relatively low and is determined by other factors, especially the severity of left ventricular impairment.

If VF or pulseless VT occurs in the context of non-ST segment elevation ACS, there may be a continuing risk of further ventricular arrhythmia. If the arrhythmia has been caused by severe myocardial ischaemia, very urgent revascularisation is needed to prevent recurrence of the ischaemia and reduce the risk of resulting arrhythmia. If this is not achievable or if the arrhythmia has occurred without evidence of severe ischaemia, the patient will be at risk of recurrent ventricular arrhythmia and should be referred to a cardiologist with a view to insertion of an implantable cardioverter-defibrillator (ICD) **before discharge from hospital.**

Patients who develop VF or pulseless VT as a late complication after myocardial infarction, or outside the context of an ACS, will be at risk of recurrent cardiac arrest and should be seen urgently by a cardiologist with a view to ICD implantation **before discharge from hospital.**

## Other complications of ACS

### Heart failure

Patients with heart failure complicating AMI or other ACS are at increased risk of deterioration, cardiac arrest and death: prompt, effective treatment of the heart failure is required to reduce risk. Give a loop diuretic (e.g., furosemide) and/or glyceryl trinitrate (sublingual and/or intravenous) for immediate symptomatic treatment. Give regular loop diuretic to maintain symptom control but review the need for this and the dose at least daily for the first few days. Ensure that ACEI treatment has been started and increase the dose as tolerated, until the target dose is achieved. In patients intolerant of ACE inhibition, consider an angiotensin receptor blocker. If LV systolic impairment is confirmed (ejection fraction 40% or less) start an aldosterone antagonist (e.g., eplerenone or spironolactone).

### Cardiogenic shock

This consists of severe hypotension with poor peripheral perfusion, often accompanied by pulmonary oedema, drowsiness or mental confusion due to poor cerebral under-perfusion and oliguria caused by poor renal perfusion. The mortality is very high, but can be reduced by early revascularisation by PCI.

Some patients may improve with inotropic therapy (e.g., dobutamine) but this requires initiation and supervision by those experienced in its use. Other treatments such as intra-aortic balloon pumping may be of benefit in selected patients, but require expert supervision.

When cardiogenic shock develops in a patient after STEMI, seek early expert assessment with a view to possible emergency PCI as this may be life-saving for some patients in this setting.

### Other cardiac arrhythmia

The treatment of other cardiac arrhythmia will be covered in more detail in Chapter 12.

When atrial fibrillation occurs in the context of an ACS it usually indicates some degree of left ventricular failure: treatment should address that as well as focusing on control of heart rate or rhythm.

When AV block occurs in the context of acute inferior wall myocardial infarction there is often excess vagal activity. QRS complexes are often narrow and heart rates may not be excessively slow. Treat symptomatic bradycardia in this setting with atropine and consider temporary cardiac pacing only if bradycardia and hypotension persist after atropine therapy. Complete AV block in this setting is usually transient and permanent cardiac pacing is hardly ever necessary.

When AV block occurs in the context of acute anterior myocardial infarction this usually implies extensive myocardial injury and a poor prognosis. The QRS complexes are usually broad and the heart rate is usually slow and resistant to atropine. Temporary cardiac pacing is usually needed and should not be delayed. Many, but not all, of those who survive this situation will require a permanent pacemaker.

## Cardiac rehabilitation

In all patients after an ACS, an effective programme of cardiac rehabilitation can speed the return to normal activity and encourage measures that will reduce future risk (see below). There is evidence that effective cardiac rehabilitation reduces the need for readmission to hospital. Cardiac rehabilitation is a continuous process, beginning in the cardiac care unit and progressing through to a community-based approach to lifestyle modification and secondary prevention.

## Secondary prevention

In patients with established coronary disease, general measures to reduce cardiovascular risk ('secondary prevention') can reduce the likelihood of future coronary events (including sudden cardiac death) and stroke.

**ALS**

## Anti-thrombotic therapy

Continued anti-platelet prophylaxis is appropriate in all patients. The majority should receive low-dose aspirin (75 mg daily). Give clopidogrel 75 mg daily (after an initial loading dose of at least 300 mg) to all patients with high-risk ACS and all those undergoing PCI. Current guidelines recommend treatment for a minimum of one year. Clopidogrel alone may be used in patients who are intolerant of aspirin. In patients who develop atrial fibrillation as a complication of ischaemic heart disease, there is an additional risk of thromboembolism from the left atrium. Warfarin is more effective than aspirin in preventing intra-cardiac thrombus formation, and should be considered in addition to, or instead of, anti-platelet therapy.

## Preservation of left ventricular function

Prognosis after AMI is determined partly by the severity of left ventricular impairment that results. Treatment after AMI with an ACEI can reduce the re-modelling that contributes to left ventricular dilatation and impairment, and where there is left ventricular systolic impairment, the use of ACEI therapy in adequate dose can reduce the risk and severity of subsequent heart failure, and the risk of future AMI and death. Echocardiographic examination of left ventricular function is appropriate during the first few days after an ACS to assess risk and identify those patients likely to benefit most from this treatment. The majority of patients should be considered for ACEI treatment during the first few days after AMI.

## Reduction of cholesterol

Further reduction in risk can be achieved by effective suppression of cholesterol concentration in the blood; specifically, suppression of LDL cholesterol. Statins reduce the risk of most future coronary events by approximately 30%. A low-fat, high-fibre diet and regular exercise will complement cholesterol suppression by drugs.

## Avoidance of smoking

At least as important in reducing risk, is the removal of other avoidable risk factors such as smoking. Information, encouragement and support for patients to help them to stop smoking should begin at an early stage after presentation with an ACS.

## Anti-hypertensive treatment

Effective control of raised blood pressure, using drugs as well as non-pharmacological methods, reduces the risk of stroke and of heart failure and contributes to some reduction in the risk of future coronary events.

## Key learning points

- The acute coronary syndromes comprise unstable angina, non-ST segment elevation myocardial infarction, and ST segment elevation myocardial infarction.

- Give oxygen, nitroglycerine, aspirin and morphine to patients presenting with acute coronary syndromes.

- Rapid initial assessment using the history, examination and 12-lead ECG will help to determine the diagnosis and immediate risk.

- Consider immediate reperfusion therapy in those patients with acute myocardial infarction accompanied by ST segment elevation or new LBBB.

- Effective assessment and immediate treatment of patients with acute coronary syndromes will reduce the risk of cardiac arrest and death.

## Further reading

International Liaison Committee on Resuscitation. Part 5. Acute Coronary Syndromes. 2005 International Consensus on Cardiopulmonary Resuscitation and Emergency Cardiovascular Care Science with Treatment Recommendations. Resuscitation 2005;67:249-69.

Arntz H-R, Bossaert L. European Resuscitation Council Guidelines for Resuscitation 2005. Section 5: Initial management of acute coronary syndromes. Resuscitation 2005;67 Suppl 1:S87-96.

Bertrand M E et al. The Task Force on the Management of Acute Coronary Syndromes of the European Society of Cardiology. Management of acute coronary syndromes presenting without persistent ST-segment elevation. European Heart Journal 2002;23:1809-40.

Van de Werf et al. The Task Force on the Management of Acute Myocardial Infarction of the European Society of Cardiology. Management of acute myocardial infarction presenting with ST-segment elevation. European Heart Journal 2003;24:28-66.

Silber S, Albertsson P, Aviles FF, et al. The Task Force for Percutaneous Coronary Interventions of the European Society of Cardiology. Guidelines for Percutaneous Coronary Interventions. European Heart Journal 2005;26:804-47.

Fox K A A et al. British Cardiac Society Working Group on the definition of myocardial infarction. Heart 2004;90:603-9.

ALS

ALS

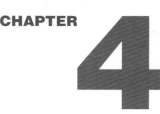
# In-hospital Resuscitation

## Objectives

To understand:

▶ **How to start resuscitation in hospital.**

▶ **How to continue resuscitation until more experienced help arrives.**

## Introduction

After in-hospital cardiac arrest, the division between basic life support and advanced life support is arbitrary; in practice, the resuscitation process is a continuum and is based on common sense. The public expect that clinical staff can undertake cardiopulmonary resuscitation (CPR). For all in-hospital cardiac arrests, ensure that:

- cardiorespiratory arrest is recognised immediately;

- help is summoned using a standard telephone number, e.g., 2222 in the UK;

- CPR is started immediately using airway adjuncts, e.g., a pocket mask, and, if indicated, defibrillation is attempted as soon as possible (within 3 min at the most).

## Why is in-hospital resuscitation different?

The exact sequence of actions after in-hospital cardiac arrest depends on several factors including:

- location (clinical/non clinical area; monitored/unmonitored area);

- skills of the first responders;

- number of responders;

- equipment available;

- hospital response system to cardiac arrest and medical emergencies, e.g., medical emergency team (MET), resuscitation team.

## Location

In patients who are being monitored closely, cardiorespiratory arrest is usually identified rapidly. Patients in many areas without facilities for close monitoring may have had a period of deterioration and may have an unwitnessed arrest. Ideally, all patients who are at high risk of cardiac arrest should be cared for in a monitored area where facilities for immediate resuscitation are available. Patients, visitors or staff may also suffer from cardiac arrest in non-clinical areas (e.g., car parks, corridors).

## Training of first responders

All healthcare professionals should be able to recognise cardiac arrest, call for help and start resuscitation. Staff should do what they have been trained to do. For example, staff in critical care and emergency medicine may have more advanced resuscitation skills and greater experience in resuscitation than those who are not involved regularly in resuscitation in their normal clinical role. Hospital staff who respond to a cardiac arrest may have different levels of skill to manage the airway, breathing and circulation. Rescuers must use the skills for which they are trained.

## Number of responders

The single responder must always ensure that help is coming. Usually, other staff are nearby and several actions can be undertaken simultaneously.

## Equipment available

Staff in all clinical areas should have immediate access to resuscitation equipment and drugs to facilitate rapid resuscitation of the patient in cardiorespiratory arrest. Ideally, the equipment used for cardiopulmonary resuscitation (including defibrillators) and the layout of equipment and drugs should be standardised throughout the hospital. You should be familiar with the resuscitation equipment used in your clinical area.

## Resuscitation team

The resuscitation team may take the form of a traditional cardiac arrest team, which is called only when cardiac arrest is recognised. Alternatively, hospitals may have strategies to recognise patients at risk of cardiac arrest and summon a team (e.g., MET) before cardiac arrest occurs. The term resuscitation team reflects the range of response teams. In-hospital cardiac arrests are rarely sudden or unexpected. A strategy of recognising patients at risk of cardiac arrest may enable some of these arrests to be prevented or prevent futile resuscitation attempts in those who are unlikely to benefit from CPR (Chapter 2).

## Sequence for collapsed patient in a hospital

An algorithm for the initial management of in-hospital cardiac arrest is shown in Figure 4.1.

### 1. Ensure personal safety

There are relatively few reports of rescuers suffering adverse effects from undertaking CPR.

- Your personal safety and that of resuscitation team members is the first priority during any resuscitation attempt.

- Check that the patient's surroundings are safe.

## In-hospital resuscitation

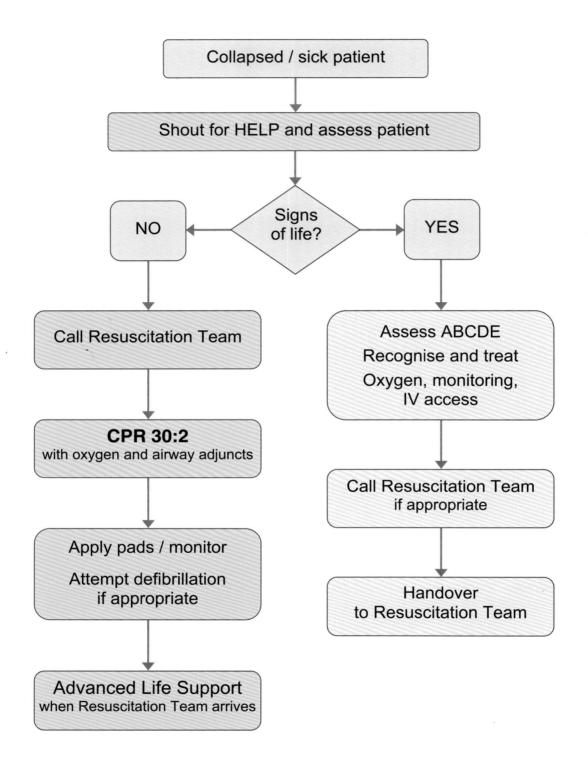

**Figure 4.1** In-hospital resuscitation

ALS

- Put on gloves as soon as possible. Other protective measures, such as eye protection, aprons and face masks, may be necessary.

- The risk of infection is much lower than perceived. There are isolated reports of infections such as tuberculosis (TB), and severe acute respiratory distress syndrome (SARS). Transmission of HIV during CPR has never been reported. Use a pocket mask with filter, or a barrier device with one-way valve to minimise infection risk during rescue breathing. The efficacy of face shields is unproved and they do not reliably prevent transmission of bacteria to the rescuer side of the shield.

- Wear full personal protective equipment (PPE) when the victim has a serious infection such as TB or SARS.

- For the latest guidance for PPE and infection see www.hpa.org.uk

- Be careful with sharps; a sharps box must be available. Use safe handling techniques for moving victims during resuscitation.

- Take care with patients exposed to poisons. Avoid mouth-to-mouth ventilation and exhaled air in hydrogen cyanide or hydrogen sulphide poisoning.

- Avoid contact with corrosive chemicals (e.g., strong acids, alkalis, paraquat) or substances such as organophosphates that are easily absorbed through the skin or respiratory tract.

- There are no reports of infection acquired during CPR training. Nevertheless, take sensible precautions to minimise potential cross-infection from manikins. Clean manikins regularly and disinfect thoroughly after each use. Some manikins have disposable face pieces and airways to simplify cleaning.

## 2. Check the patient for a response

- If you see a patient collapse or find a patient apparently unconscious in a clinical area first shout for help, then assess if he is responsive (shake and shout). Gently shake his shoulders and ask loudly: "Are you all right?" (Figure 4.2).

- If other members of staff are nearby it will be possible to undertake actions simultaneously.

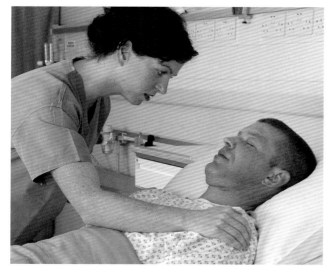

**Figure 4.2 Shake and shout**

### 3A If he responds

- Urgent medical assessment is needed. Depending on your hospital, this may take the form of a resuscitation team (e.g., MET). While awaiting the team, assess the patient using the ABCDE approach, give oxygen, attach monitoring, and obtain venous access.

### 3B If he does not respond

- The exact sequence will depend on your training and experience in assessment of breathing and circulation in sick patients. Agonal breathing (occasional gasps, slow, laboured or noisy breathing) is common in the early stages of cardiac arrest and is a sign of cardiac arrest and should not be confused as a sign of life.

- Shout for help (if not already).

- Turn the patient on to his back.

- Open the airway using head tilt and chin lift (Figure 4.3).

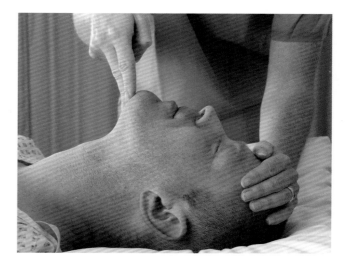

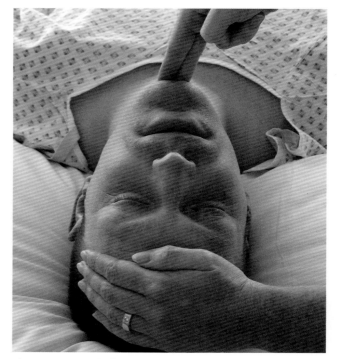

**Figure 4.3 Head tilt and chin lift**

**ALS**

- Look in the mouth. If a foreign body or debris is visible, remove this with forceps or suction.

- If there is a risk of cervical spine injury, establish a clear upper airway by using jaw thrust or chin lift in combination with manual in-line stabilisation (MILS) of the head and neck by an assistant (if enough personnel are available). If life threatening airway obstruction persists despite effective application of jaw thrust or chin lift, add head tilt a small amount at a time until the airway is open; establishing a patent airway takes priority over concerns about a potential cervical spine injury.

- Keeping the airway open, look, listen, and feel for no more than **10 sec** (Figure 4.4) to determine if the

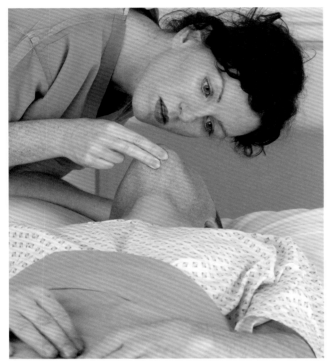

**Figure 4.4 Looking for breathing and any other movement**

victim is breathing normally (an occasional gasp, slow, laboured or noisy breathing is not normal) or has other signs of life.

  - Look for chest movement (breathing or coughing).

  - Look for any other movement or signs of life.

  - Listen at the victim's mouth for breath sounds.

  - Feel for air on your cheek.

- If the patient has no signs of life (based on lack of movement, breathing, coughing), start CPR until more experienced help arrives or the patient shows signs of life.

- If trained and experienced in the assessment of sick patients, check for breathing and assess the carotid pulse at the same time (Figure 4.5).

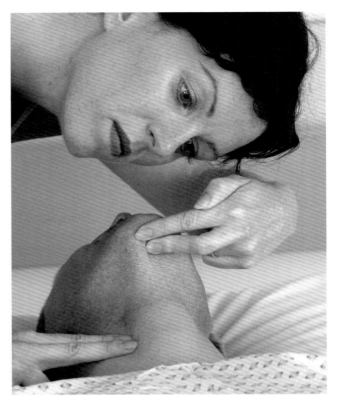

**Figure 4.5 Simultaneous check for breathing and carotid pulse**

- If the patient has no signs of life, no pulse, or if there is any doubt, start CPR immediately.

- If unsure, do not delay starting CPR. Delays in diagnosis of cardiac arrest and starting CPR will effect survival adversely and must be avoided. Starting CPR on a very sick patient with a low cardiac output is unlikely to be harmful and may be beneficial.

- Assess the patient to confirm cardiac arrest even if the patient is monitored in a critical care area.

## 4A If he has a pulse or signs of life

- Urgent medical assessment is required. Depending on the local protocols, this may take the form of a resuscitation team. While awaiting this team, assess the patient using the ABCDE approach, give oxygen, attach monitoring, and insert an intravenous cannula.

## 4B If there is no pulse or signs of life

- Start CPR and get a colleague to call the resuscitation team (Figure 4.6) and collect the resuscitation equipment and a defibrillator.

**ALS**

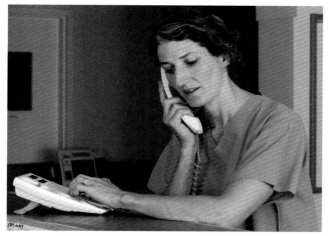

**Figure 4.6 Call the resuscitation team**

- If alone, leave the patient to get help and equipment.

- Give 30 chest compressions followed by 2 ventilations.

- The correct hand position for chest compression is the middle of the lower half of the sternum (Figure 4.7).

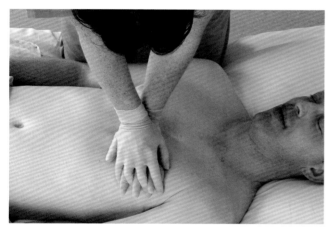

**Figure 4.7 Hand position for chest compressions**

- This hand position can be found quickly if you have been taught to 'place the heel of one hand in the centre of the chest with the other hand on top' and your teaching included a demonstration of placing hands in the middle of the lower half of the sternum (Figure 4.8).

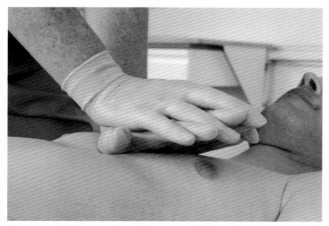

**Figure 4.8 Hands placed in the middle of the lower half of the sternum**

- Compress to a depth of 4-5 cm and at a rate of 100 compressions min$^{-1}$. Allow the chest to recoil completely after each compression. Take approximately the same amount of time for compression and relaxation.

- Each time compressions are resumed, place your hands without delay in the centre of the chest.

- Do not rely on a palpable carotid or femoral pulse to assess effective arterial flow.

- Use whatever equipment is available immediately for airway and ventilation. A pocket mask, which can be supplemented with an oral airway should be readily available (Figure 4.9). Alternatively, use a laryngeal mask airway and self-inflating bag, or bag-mask, according to local policy. Attempt tracheal intubation only if trained and competent to do so.

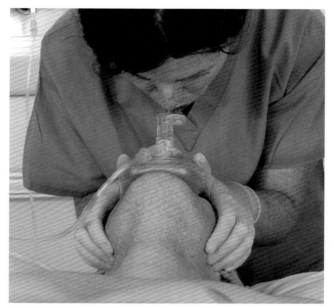

**Figure 4.9 Use of the pocket mask**

- Use an inspiratory time of about 1 sec and give enough volume to produce a visible chest rise. Add supplemental oxygen as soon as possible.

- Avoid rapid or forceful breaths.

- Once the patient's trachea has been intubated, continue chest compressions uninterrupted (except for defibrillation or pulse checks when indicated), at a rate of 100 min$^{-1}$, and ventilate the lungs at approximately 10 breaths min$^{-1}$. Avoid hyperventilation.

- If airway and ventilation equipment are unavailable, give mouth-to-mouth ventilation. If there are clinical reasons to avoid mouth-to-mouth contact, or you are unwilling or unable to do this, do chest compressions until help or airway equipment arrives. A pocket mask should be immediately available in all clinical areas.

- When the defibrillator arrives, apply the electrodes to the patient and analyse the rhythm. Self-adhesive electrode pads or a 'quick-look' paddles technique (Figure 4.10) will enable faster assessment of heart rhythm than attaching ECG electrodes.

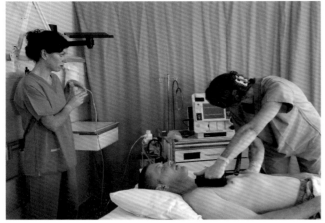

**Figure 4.10 'Quick-look' technique with defibrillator paddles**

- If self-adhesive defibrillation pads are available, and there is more than one rescuer, apply the pads without interrupting chest compressions (Figure 4.11). Pause briefly to assess the heart rhythm. If indicated, attempt manual defibrillation. Alternatively follow the automated external defibrillator (AED) voice prompts.

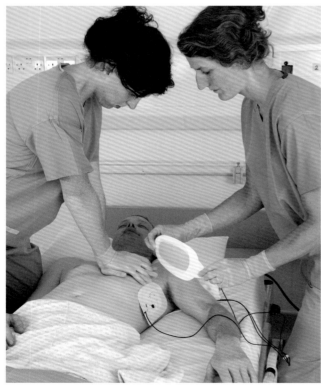

**Figure 4.11 Maintain chest compressions while self-adhesive pads are applied**

- Restart chest compressions immediately after the defibrillation attempt. Do not pause to assess the pulse or heart rhythm. Minimise interruptions to chest compressions.

- Continue resuscitation until the resuscitation team arrives or the patient shows signs of life. Follow the voice prompts if using an AED.

- If you are using a manual defibrillator, follow the algorithm for advanced life support (Chapter 5).

- Once resuscitation is under way, and if there are sufficient people, prepare intravenous cannulae and drugs likely to be used by the resuscitation team (e.g., adrenaline).

- Identify one person to be responsible for handover to the resuscitation team leader. Locate the patient's records.

- The person doing chest compressions will get tired. If there are enough rescuers, this person should change about every 2 min.

- The quality of chest compressions during in-hospital CPR is often poor. Guide or, if necessary, change the person doing chest compressions if this is the case.

- Use a watch or clock for timing between defibrillation attempts. It is difficult to keep track of the number of 30:2 cycles.

## 4C If he is not breathing and has a pulse (respiratory arrest)

- Ventilate the patient's lungs (as described above) and check for a circulation every 10 breaths (about every minute).

- This diagnosis can be made only if you are confident in assessing breathing and pulse or the patient has other signs of life (e.g., warm and well perfused, normal capillary refill).

- If there are any doubts about the presence of a pulse, start chest compressions until more experienced help arrives.

- All patients in respiratory arrest will develop cardiac arrest if the respiratory arrest is not treated rapidly and effectively.

## 5 If the patient has a monitored and witnessed cardiac arrest

- Confirm cardiac arrest and shout for help.

- Give a precordial thump (Chapter 5) if the rhythm is ventricular fibrillation/pulseless ventricular tachycardia (VF/VT) and a defibrillator is not available for immediate delivery of a shock.

- If the initial rhythm is VF/VT and a defibrillator is available for immediate shock delivery, give a shock.

- Start CPR immediately after the shock is delivered as described above.

## Key learning points

- The exact sequence of actions after in-hospital cardiac arrest depends on the location, skills of the first responders, number of responders, equipment available, and the hospital response system to cardiac arrest and medical emergencies.

- Safety of the resuscitation team is the first priority during any resuscitation attempt.

- Minimise interruptions to chest compressions.

## Further reading

International Liaison Committee on Resuscitation. Part 4. Advanced Life Support. 2005 International Consensus on Cardiopulmonary Resuscitation and Emergency Cardiovascular Care Science with Treatment Recommendations. Resuscitation 2005;67:213-47.

Nolan JP, Deakin CD, Soar J, Bottiger BW, Smith G. European Resuscitation Council Guidelines for Resuscitation 2005 Section 4: Adult advanced life support. Resuscitation 2005; 67 Suppl 1:S39-86.

Abella BS, Alvarado JP, Myklebust H, et al. Quality of cardiopulmonary resuscitation during in-hospital cardiac arrest. JAMA 2005;293:305-10.

Gabbott D, Smith G, Mitchell S, et al. Cardiopulmonary resuscitation standards for clinical practice and training in the UK. Resuscitation 2005;64:13-9.

Guidance for safer handling during resuscitation in hospitals. July 2001. Resuscitation Council UK.

Perkins GD, Stephenson B, Hulme J, Monsieurs KG. Birmingham assessment of breathing study (BABS). Resuscitation 2005;64:109-13.

Ruppert M, Reith MW, Widmann JH, et al. Checking for breathing: evaluation of the diagnostic capability of emergency medical services personnel, physicians, medical students, and medical laypersons. Ann Emerg Med 1999;34:720-9.

Handley AJ. Teaching hand placement for chest compression—a simpler technique. Resuscitation 2002;53:29-36.

Heilman KM, Muschenheim C. Primary cutaneous tuberculosis resulting from mouth-to-mouth respiration. N Engl J Med 1965;273:1035-6.

Christian MD, Loutfy M, McDonald LC, et al. Possible SARS coronavirus transmission during cardiopulmonary resuscitation. Emerg Infect Dis 2004;10:287-93.

Cydulka RK, Connor PJ, Myers TF, Pavza G, Parker M. Prevention of oral bacterial flora transmission by using mouth-to-mask ventilation during CPR. J Emerg Med 991;9:317-21.

Kern KB, Sanders AB, Raife J, Milander MM, Otto CW, Ewy GA. A study of chest compression rates during cardiopulmonary resuscitation in humans: the importanceof rate-directed chest compressions. Arch Intern Med 1992;152:145-9.

ALS

# Advanced Life Support Algorithm

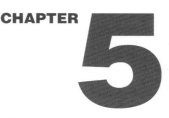

## CHAPTER 5

## Objectives

To understand:

▶ **The function of the advanced life support (ALS) algorithm.**

▶ **The treatment of ventricular fibrillation / pulseless ventricular tachycardia (VF/VT).**

▶ **The treatment of non-shockable rhythms.**

▶ **The indication and technique for giving a precordial thump.**

▶ **The potentially reversible causes of cardiac arrest.**

▶ **The role of the resuscitation team leader.**

## Introduction

Heart rhythms associated with cardiac arrest are divided into two groups: shockable rhythms (ventricular fibrillation / pulseless ventricular tachycardia (VF/VT)) and non-shockable rhythms (asystole and pulseless electrical activity (PEA)). The principle difference in the management of these two groups of arrhythmias is the need for attempted defibrillation in patients with VF/VT. Subsequent actions, including chest compressions, airway management and ventilation, venous access, administration of adrenaline and the identification and correction of reversible factors, are common to both groups.

The ALS algorithm is a standardised approach to cardiac arrest management. This has the advantage of enabling treatment to be delivered expediently, without protracted discussion. It enables each member of the cardiac arrest team to predict and prepare for the next stage in the patient's treatment, further enhancing efficiency of the team. Although the ALS algorithm (Figure 5.1) is applicable to most cardiac arrests, additional interventions may be indicated for cardiac arrest caused by special circumstances (Chapter 13).

The interventions that definitely improve survival after cardiac arrest are early defibrillation for VF/VT and prompt and effective CPR (chest compressions and ventilations). Advanced airway intervention and the delivery of drugs have not been shown to increase survival to hospital discharge after cardiac arrest, but they are still included among ALS interventions. Thus, during ALS, attention must be focused on early defibrillation and high quality, uninterrupted CPR.

## Shockable rhythms (VF/VT)

In adults, the commonest rhythm at the time of cardiac arrest is VF, which may be preceded by a period of VT, by a bradyarrhythmia, or less commonly, supraventricular tachycardia (SVT). Having confirmed cardiac arrest, summon help (including a request for a defibrillator) and start CPR, beginning with chest compressions, with a compression: ventilation ratio of 30:2 as described in the previous chapter. As soon as the defibrillator arrives apply self-adhesive pads or paddles to the chest to diagnose the rhythm. If VF/VT is confirmed, follow the treatment steps below.

## Treatment of shockable rhythms (VF/VT)

● Attempt defibrillation. Give one shock of 150-200 J biphasic (360 J monophasic).

● Immediately resume chest compressions (30:2) without reassessing the rhythm or feeling for a pulse.

● Continue CPR for 2 min, then pause briefly to check the monitor:

  – *If VF/VT persists:*

    ● Give a further (2nd) shock of 150-360 J biphasic (360 J monophasic).

    ● Resume CPR immediately and continue for 2 min.

    ● Pause briefly to check the monitor.

    ● If VF/VT persists give adrenaline 1 mg IV followed immediately by a (3rd) shock of 150-360 J biphasic (360 J monophasic).

    ● Resume CPR immediately and continue for 2 min.

    ● Pause briefly to check the monitor.

    ● If VF/VT persists give amiodarone 300 mg IV followed immediately by a (4th) shock of 150-360 J biphasic (360 J monophasic).

    ● Resume CPR immediately and continue for 2 min.

    ● Give adrenaline 1 mg IV immediately before alternate shocks (i.e., approximately every 3-5 min).

    ● Give further shocks after each 2 min period of CPR and after confirming that VF/VT persists.

  – *If organised electrical activity compatible with a cardiac output is seen, check for a pulse:*

    ● If a pulse is present, start post-resuscitation care.

    ● If no pulse is present, continue CPR and switch to the non-shockable algorithm.

  – *If asystole is seen, continue CPR and switch to the non-shockable algorithm.*

## Adult Advanced Life Support Algorithm

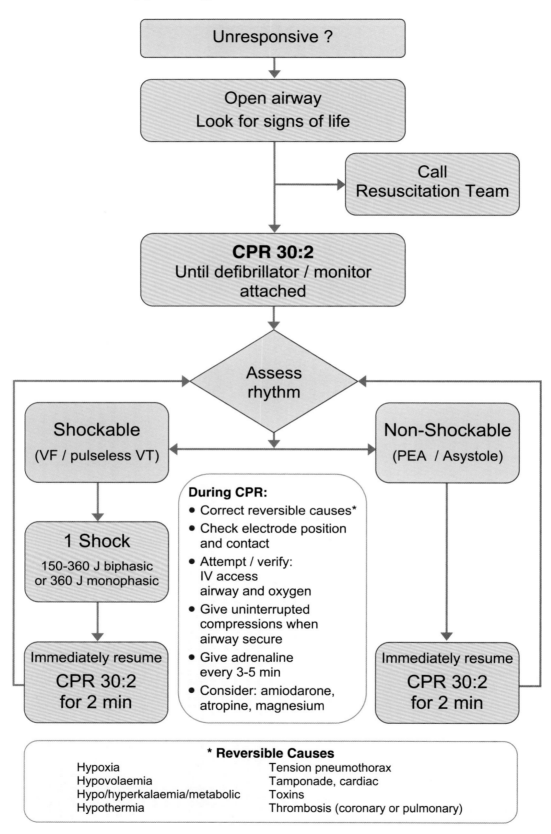

**Figure 5.1 Adult Advanced Life Support Algorithm**

The interval between stopping compressions and delivering a shock must be minimised and certainly should not exceed 10 sec. Longer interruptions to chest compressions reduce the chance of a shock restoring a spontaneous circulation

Chest compressions are resumed immediately after a shock without checking the rhythm or a pulse because even if the defibrillation attempt is successful in restoring a perfusing rhythm, it is very rare for a pulse to be palpable immediately after defibrillation and the delay in trying to palpate a pulse will further compromise the myocardium if a perfusing rhythm has not been restored. If a perfusing rhythm has been restored, giving chest compressions does not increase the chance of VF recurring. In the presence of post-shock asystole chest compressions may usefully induce VF.

The first dose of adrenaline is given immediately after confirmation of the rhythm and just before delivery of the third shock (**drug–shock–CPR–rhythm check** sequence); subsequent doses of adrenaline are given just before alternate shocks for as long as VF/VT persists. Have the adrenaline ready to give, so that the delay between stopping chest compressions and delivery of the shock is minimised. The adrenaline that is given immediately before the shock will be circulated by the CPR that immediately follows the shock. Do not delay giving a shock to wait for adrenaline - if the adrenaline is not ready in time, give it after delivery of the shock.

During CPR, adrenaline is given every 3-5 min. When switching from the non-shockable to the shockable side of the algorithm, the next dose of adrenaline will be given before the first or the second shock depending on when adrenaline was last given.

When the rhythm is checked 2 min after giving a shock, if a non-shockable rhythm is present and the rhythm is organised (complexes appear regular or narrow), try to palpate a pulse. Rhythm checks must be brief, and pulse checks undertaken only if an organised rhythm is observed. If an organised rhythm is seen during a 2 min period of CPR, do not interrupt chest compressions to palpate a pulse unless the patient shows signs of life suggesting return of spontaneous circulation (ROSC). If there is any doubt about the presence of a pulse in the presence of an organised rhythm, resume CPR. If the patient has ROSC, begin post-resuscitation care. If the patient's rhythm changes to asystole or PEA, see non-shockable rhythms below.

There is no evidence that giving any anti-arrhythmic drug routinely during human cardiac arrest increases survival to hospital discharge. In comparison with placebo and lidocaine, the use of amiodarone in shock-refractory VF improves the short-term outcome of survival to hospital admission. Lidocaine 100 mg IV (or 1-1.5 mg kg$^{-1}$) may be used as an alternative if amiodarone is not available, but do not give lidocaine if amiodarone has been given already. Give magnesium (2g IV bolus) for shock-refractory VF if there is any possibility of hypomagnesaemia (e.g., patient treated with diuretic). It is important in shock-refractory VF/VT to check the electrode/defibrillating paddle positions

and contacts, and the adequacy of the coupling medium, e.g., gel pads. The duration of any individual resuscitation attempt is a matter of clinical judgement, and should take into account the perceived prospect of a successful outcome. If it was considered appropriate to start resuscitation, it is usually considered worthwhile continuing as long as the patient remains in identifiable VF/VT.

If there is doubt about whether the rhythm is asystole or very fine VF, do not attempt defibrillation; instead, continue chest compressions and ventilation. Very fine VF that is difficult to distinguish from asystole is unlikely to be shocked successfully into a perfusing rhythm. Continuing good quality CPR may improve the amplitude and frequency of the VF and improve the chance of subsequent successful defibrillation to a perfusing rhythm. Delivering repeated shocks in an attempt to defibrillate what is thought to be very fine VF will increase myocardial injury both directly from the electric current and indirectly from the interruptions in coronary blood flow. If the rhythm is clearly VF, attempt defibrillation.

## Precordial thump

Consider giving a single precordial thump when VF/VT cardiac arrest is confirmed rapidly after a witnessed and monitored, sudden collapse if a defibrillator is not to hand immediately. The precordial thump should be given only by healthcare professionals trained in the technique.

Using the ulnar edge of a tightly clenched fist, deliver a sharp impact to the lower half of the sternum from a height of about 20 cm, then retract the fist immediately to create an impulse-like stimulus (Figure 5.2). A precordial thump is most likely to be successful in converting VT to sinus rhythm. Successful treatment of VF by precordial thump is much less likely: in all the reported successful cases the precordial thump was given within the first 10 seconds of VF (Figure 5.3). There are very rare reports of a precordial thump converting a perfusing to a non-perfusing rhythm.

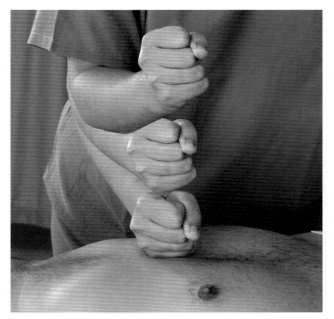

**Figure 5.2 Precordial thump**

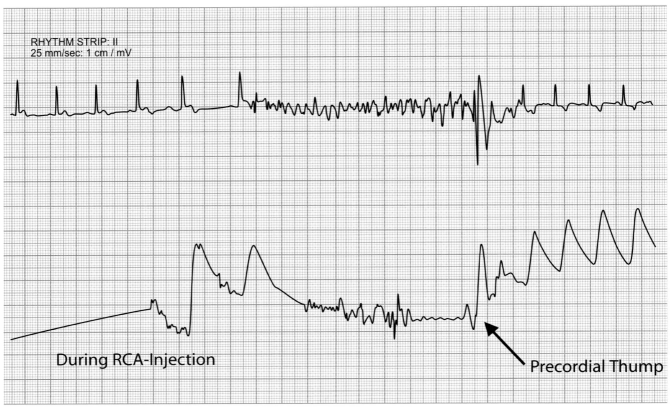

**Figure 5.3 VF occurring during coronary angiography. A single precordial thump terminates the VF. The lower trace represents the pressure in the right coronary artery (RCA).**

# Non-shockable rhythms (PEA and asystole)

Pulseless electrical activity (PEA) is defined as organised cardiac electrical activity in the absence of any palpable pulses. These patients often have some mechanical myocardial contractions but they are too weak to produce a detectable pulse or blood pressure. PEA may be caused by reversible conditions that can be treated (see below). Survival following cardiac arrest with asystole or PEA is unlikely unless a reversible cause can be found and treated quickly and effectively.

## Treatment for PEA

- Start CPR 30:2.

- Give adrenaline 1 mg IV as soon as intravascular access is achieved.

- Continue CPR 30:2 until the airway is secured - then continue chest compressions without pausing during ventilation.

- Recheck the rhythm after 2 min:

  - *If organised electrical activity is seen, check for a pulse and/or signs of life:*

    - If a pulse and/or signs of life are present, start post resuscitation care.

    - If no pulse and/or no signs of life are present (PEA):

      - Continue CPR.

- Recheck the rhythm after 2 min and proceed accordingly.

- Give further adrenaline 1 mg IV every 3-5 min (alternate loops).

- *If VF/VT at rhythm check, change to shockable side of algorithm.*

- *If asystole or an agonal rhythm seen at rhythm check:*

  - Continue CPR.

  - Recheck the rhythm after 2 min and proceed accordingly.

  - Give further adrenaline 1 mg IV every 3-5 min (alternate loops).

## Treatment for asystole and slow PEA (rate < 60 min$^{-1}$)

- Start CPR 30:2.

- Check that the leads are attached correctly without stopping CPR.

- Give adrenaline 1 mg IV as soon as intravascular access is achieved.

- Give atropine 3 mg IV (once only).

- Continue CPR 30:2 until the airway is secured; then continue chest compressions without pausing during ventilation.

- Recheck the rhythm after 2 min and proceed accordingly.

**ALS**

- If VF/VT recurs, change to the shockable rhythm algorithm.

- Give adrenaline 1 mg IV every 3-5 min (alternate loops).

### Asystole

Asystole is a condition that could be exacerbated or precipitated by excessive vagal discharge. This could be reversed by a drug that blocks the effect of vagal discharge. Therefore, give atropine 3 mg (the dose that will provide maximum vagal blockade) if there is asystole or the rhythm is slow PEA (rate < 60 min$^{-1}$).

Whenever a diagnosis of asystole is made, check the ECG carefully for the presence of P waves because in this situation ventricular standstill may be treated effectively by cardiac pacing. Attempts to pace true asystole are unlikely to be successful.

# During CPR

During the treatment of persistent VF/VT or PEA / asystole, emphasis is placed on good quality chest compressions between defibrillation attempts, recognising and treating reversible causes (4 Hs and 4 Ts), obtaining a secure airway, and intravenous access.

During CPR with a 30:2 ratio the underlying rhythm may be seen clearly on the monitor as compressions are paused to enable ventilation. If VF is seen during this brief pause (whether on the shockable or non-shockable side of the algorithm), do not attempt defibrillation at this stage; instead, continue with CPR until the 2 min period is completed. Knowing that the rhythm is VF, the team should be fully prepared to deliver a shock with minimal delay at the end of the 2 min period of CPR.

The quality of chest compressions and ventilations are important determinants of outcome, yet are frequently performed poorly by healthcare professionals. Providing CPR with a ratio of 30:2 is tiring. As soon as the airway is secured, continue chest compressions without pausing during ventilation. To reduce fatigue, change the individual undertaking compressions every 2 min.

## Airway and ventilation

Tracheal intubation provides the most reliable airway but should be attempted only if the healthcare provider is properly trained and has adequate ongoing experience with the technique. Personnel skilled in intubation should attempt laryngoscopy without stopping chest compressions - a brief pause in chest compressions may be required as the tube is passed through the vocal cords. Alternatively, to avoid any interruptions in chest compressions, the intubation attempt may be deferred until return of spontaneous circulation. No intubation attempt should take longer than 30 sec: if intubation has not been achieved after this time, recommence bag-mask ventilation. After intubation, confirm correct tube position and secure the tube. Once the patient's trachea has been intubated, continue chest compressions, at a rate of 100 min$^{-1}$,

without pausing during ventilation. Ventilate the lungs at 10 breaths min$^{-1}$. It is important not to hyperventilate the patient. A pause in the chest compressions allows the coronary perfusion pressure to fall substantially. On resuming compressions there is some delay before the original coronary perfusion pressure is restored, thus, chest compressions uninterrupted for ventilation produce a substantially higher mean coronary perfusion pressure.

In the absence of personnel skilled in tracheal intubation, acceptable alternatives are the Combitube, laryngeal mask airway (LMA), ProSeal LMA, or Laryngeal Tube (Chapter 6). Once one of these airways has been inserted, attempt to deliver continuous chest compressions, uninterrupted during ventilation. If excessive gas leakage results in inadequate ventilation of the patient's lungs, chest compressions will have to be interrupted to enable ventilation.

## Intravenous access

Obtain intravenous access if this has not been done already. Although peak drug concentrations are higher and circulation times are shorter when drugs are injected into a central venous catheter compared with a peripheral cannula, insertion of a central venous catheter requires interruption of CPR and is associated with several potential complications. Peripheral venous cannulation is quicker, easier, and safer. Drugs injected peripherally must be followed by a flush of at least 20 ml of fluid and elevation of the extremity for 10-20 sec to facilitate drug delivery to the central circulation. Alternative routes such as the intraosseous or tracheal routes are discussed in Chapter 9.

## Reversible causes

Potential causes or aggravating factors for which specific treatment exists must be considered during any cardiac arrest. For ease of memory, these are divided into two groups of four based upon their initial letter — either H or T. More details on many of these conditions are covered in Chapter 13.

- Hypoxia

- Hypovolaemia

- Hyperkalaemia, hypokalaemia, hypoglycaemia, hypocalcaemia, acidaemia and other metabolic disorders

- Hypothermia

- Tension pneumothorax

- Tamponade

- Toxins

- Thrombosis (pulmonary embolism or coronary thrombosis)

### The four Hs

Minimise the risk of **hypoxia** by ensuring that the patient's lungs are ventilated adequately with 100% oxygen. Make sure there is adequate chest rise and bilateral breath sounds.

Using the techniques described in Chapter 6, check carefully that the tracheal tube is not misplaced in a bronchus or the oesophagus.

Pulseless electrical activity caused by **hypovolaemia** is due usually to severe haemorrhage. This may be precipitated by trauma (Chapter 13), gastrointestinal bleeding, or rupture of an aortic aneurysm. Intravascular volume should be restored rapidly with fluid, coupled with urgent surgery to stop the haemorrhage.

**Hyperkalaemia,** hypokalaemia, hypoglycaemia, hypocalcaemia, acidaemia and other metabolic disorders are detected by biochemical tests or suggested by the patient's medical history e.g., renal failure (Chapter 13). A 12-lead ECG may show suggestive features. Intravenous calcium chloride is indicated in the presence of hyperkalaemia, hypocalcaemia, and calcium channel-blocker overdose.

Suspect **hypothermia** in any drowning incident (Chapter 13); use a low reading thermometer.

### The four Ts

A **tension pneumothorax** may be the primary cause of PEA and may follow attempts at central venous catheter insertion. The diagnosis is made clinically. Decompress rapidly by needle thoracocentesis, and then insert a chest drain.

Cardiac **tamponade** is difficult to diagnose because the typical signs of distended neck veins and hypotension cannot be assessed during cardiac arrest. Cardiac arrest after penetrating chest trauma should raise strong suspicion of tamponade - the need for needle pericardiocentesis or resuscitative thoracotomy should be considered in this setting (Chapter 13).

In the absence of a specific history of accidental or deliberate ingestion, poisoning by therapeutic or **toxic** substances may be difficult to detect but in some cases may be revealed later by laboratory investigations (Chapter 13). Where available, the appropriate antidotes should be used but most often the required treatment is supportive. The commonest cause of **thromboembolic** or mechanical circulatory obstruction is massive pulmonary embolism. If cardiac arrest is thought to be caused by pulmonary embolism consider giving a thrombolytic drug immediately.

### Signs of life

If signs of life (such as regular respiratory effort, movement) or readings from patient monitors compatible with ROSC (e.g., exhaled carbon dioxide, arterial blood pressure) appear during CPR, stop CPR briefly and check the monitor. If an organised rhythm is present, check for a pulse. If a pulse is palpable, continue post-resuscitation care and/or treatment of peri-arrest arrhythmias if appropriate. If no pulse is present, continue CPR.

## The resuscitation team

The resuscitation team may take the form of a traditional cardiac arrest team, which is called only when cardiac arrest is recognised. Alternatively, hospitals may have strategies to recognise patients at risk of cardiac arrest and summon a team (e.g., medical emergency team) before cardiac arrest occurs (Chapter 2). The term resuscitation team reflects the range of response teams.

The composition of the team with responsibility for the resuscitation of patients in cardiopulmonary arrest will vary from centre to centre but should reflect the competencies required during a resuscitation attempt. These include airway interventions, including tracheal intubation; intravenous cannulation, including central venous access; defibrillation (advisory and manual) and cardioversion; drug administration; the ability to undertake advanced resuscitation skills (e.g., external cardiac pacing, pericardiocentesis); and skills required for post-resuscitation care.

The resuscitation team leader must be identified early in the resuscitation attempt. The team leader should be ALS trained and is usually one of the doctors on the resuscitation team. The team leader is responsible for directing and co-ordinating the resuscitation attempt, and is responsible for safety at the cardiopulmonary arrest. The team leader is responsible for ending the resuscitation attempt when indicated. After the resuscitation attempt, the team leader is responsible for documentation (including audit forms) and for communication with relatives and other healthcare professionals involved in the patient's management.

**The team leader should:**

1. State early on that they are assuming the role of team leader.

2. Follow recognised resuscitation guidelines or explain a reason for any significant deviation from standard protocols.

3. Maintain a calm and positive attitude; encourage and support team members.

4. Make decisions confidently and quickly. If you are unsure, consult with the team, be flexible but then give clear directions. Call for senior advice and assistance if appropriate.

5. Play to the strengths of team members and allow them some autonomy if their skills are adequate.

6. Allocate roles and tasks throughout the resuscitation and be specific. This avoids several people or nobody attempting the task!

7. Give clear, precise directions throughout the resuscitation attempt.

8. Plan ahead and inform the team of anticipated requirements.

9. Maintain realistic performance standards without being critical.

10. Try to stand back, allocate tasks to team members and maintain an overview.

11. At the end of the resuscitation attempt, thank the team and ensure that staff and relatives are being supported. Complete all documentation and ensure an adequate handover.

**The resuscitation team members should:**

1. Appoint a team leader as soon as possible.

2. Follow the team leader's instructions.

3. Contribute ideas and suggestions through the team leader.

4. Be clear and precise when passing on information but keep the general noise levels down.

5. Where appropriate work autonomously following guidelines and anticipating requirements.

6. Ask for assistance if you are unsure.

7. Confirm completion of an allocated task and provide essential information to the leader.

8. Support the team leader. Offer help with tasks during resuscitation and in the post resuscitation period.

## Key learning points

- The ALS algorithm provides a framework for the standardised resuscitation of all adult patients in cardiac arrest.

- Treatment depends on the underlying rhythm.

- Whenever possible, secure the airway early to enable continuous chest compressions.

- The quality of chest compression and ventilation is an important determinant of outcome.

- Look for reversible causes and, if present, treat early.

- The resuscitation team leader has an important role to play in leading the resuscitation team.

## Further reading

International Liaison Committee on Resuscitation. Part 3. Defibrillation. 2005 International Consensus on Cardiopulmonary Resuscitation and Emergency Cardiovascular Care Science with Treatment Recommendations. Resuscitation 2005;67:203-11.

International Liaison Committee on Resuscitation. Part 4. Advanced Life Support. 2005 International Consensus on Cardiopulmonary Resuscitation and Emergency Cardiovascular Care Science with Treatment Recommendations. Resuscitation 2005;67:213-47.

Nolan JP, Deakin CD, Soar J, Bottiger BW, Smith G. European Resuscitation Council Guidelines for Resuscitation 2005. Section 4: Adult advanced life support. Resuscitation 2005;67 Suppl 1:S39-86.

Deakin CD, Nolan JP. European Resuscitation Council Guidelines for Resuscitation 2005. Section 3: Electrical therapies: automated external defibrillators, defibrillation, cardioversion and pacing. Resuscitation 2005; 67 Suppl 1:S25-37.

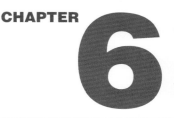

## CHAPTER 6

# Airway Management and Ventilation

## Objectives

To understand:

▶ **The causes and recognition of airway obstruction.**

▶ **Techniques for airway management when starting resuscitation.**

▶ **The use of simple adjuncts to maintain airway patency.**

▶ **The use of simple devices for ventilating the lungs.**

## Section 1. Basic airway management and ventilation

## Introduction

Patients requiring resuscitation often have an obstructed airway, usually caused by loss of consciousness, but occasionally it may be the primary cause of cardiorespiratory arrest. Prompt assessment, with control of the airway and provision of ventilation is essential. This will help to prevent secondary hypoxic damage to the brain and other vital organs. Without adequate oxygenation it may be impossible to restore an organised, perfusing rhythm.

## Causes of airway obstruction

Obstruction of the airway may be partial or complete. It may occur at any level from the nose and mouth down to the bronchi. In the unconscious patient, the commonest site of airway obstruction is at the level of the pharynx. The precise cause of airway obstruction in the unconscious state has been identified by studying patients under general anaesthesia. Airway obstruction had previously been attributed to posterior displacement of the tongue caused by decreased muscle tone, with the tongue ultimately touching the posterior pharyngeal wall. These studies of anaesthetised patients have shown that the site of airway obstruction is more often at the soft palate and epiglottis and not the tongue. Obstruction may also be caused by vomit or blood, as a result of regurgitation of gastric contents or trauma, or by foreign bodies. Laryngeal obstruction may be caused by oedema from burns, inflammation or anaphylaxis. Upper airway stimulation or inhalation of foreign material may cause laryngeal spasm. Obstruction of the airway below the larynx is less common, but may be caused by excessive bronchial secretions, mucosal oedema, bronchospasm, pulmonary oedema, or aspiration of gastric contents.

## Recognition of airway obstruction

This is best achieved by the look, listen and feel approach.

- LOOK for chest and abdominal movements.

- LISTEN and FEEL for airflow at the mouth and nose.

In partial airway obstruction, air entry is diminished and usually noisy.

- Inspiratory stridor - caused by obstruction at the laryngeal level or above.

- Expiratory wheeze - suggests obstruction of the lower airways, which tend to collapse and obstruct during expiration.

- Gurgling - suggests the presence of liquid or semisolid foreign material in the upper airways.

- Snoring - arises when the pharynx is partially occluded by the tongue or palate.

- Crowing or stridor - is the sound of laryngeal spasm or obstruction.

Complete airway obstruction in a patient who is making respiratory efforts causes paradoxical chest and abdominal movement, described as 'see-saw breathing'. As the patient attempts to breathe in, the chest is drawn in and the abdomen expands; the opposite occurs in expiration. This is in contrast to the normal breathing pattern of synchronous movement of the abdomen upwards and outwards (pushed down by the diaphragm) with lifting of the chest wall. During airway obstruction, accessory muscles of respiration are used - the neck and the shoulder muscles contract to assist movement of the thoracic cage. There may also be intercostal and subcostal recession and a tracheal tug. Full examination of the neck, chest and abdomen should enable differentiation of the movements associated with complete airway obstruction from those of normal breathing. Listen for airflow: normal breathing should be quiet, completely obstructed breathing will be silent, and noisy breathing indicates partial airway obstruction.

Unless airway obstruction can be relieved to enable adequate lung ventilation within a few minutes it will cause injury to the brain and other vital organs, and cardiac arrest. Whenever possible, give high concentration oxygen while attempting to relieve airway obstruction. As airway patency is restored, blood oxygen saturation will be restored more rapidly if the inspired oxygen concentration is high.

## Patients with tracheostomies or permanent tracheal stomas

A patient with a tracheostomy tube or a permanent tracheal stoma (usually following a laryngectomy) may develop airway obstruction from blockage of the tracheostomy tube or stoma — airway obstruction cannot occur at the level of the pharynx. Remove any foreign material from the stoma or tracheostomy tube. If necessary, remove the tracheostomy tube or, if present, exchange the tracheostomy tube liner. Apply oxygen and, if required, assist ventilation via the stoma or tracheostomy tube, and not the mouth.

# Basic techniques for opening the airway

Once airway obstruction is recognised, take immediate action to relieve the obstruction and maintain a clear airway. Three manoeuvres that can be used to relieve upper airway obstruction are:

- head tilt;

- chin lift;

- jaw thrust.

## Head tilt and chin lift

Place one hand on the patient's forehead and tilt the head back gently; place the fingertips of the other hand under the point of the patient's chin, and gently lift to stretch the anterior neck structures (Figure 6.1).

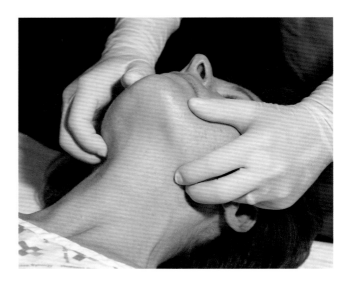

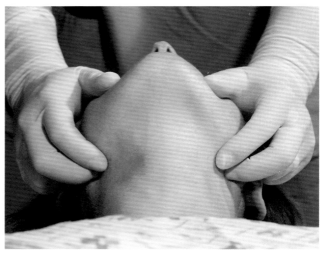

**Figure 6.2 Jaw thrust**

### Procedure for jaw thrust

- Identify the angle of the mandible.

- With the index and other fingers placed behind the angle of the mandible, apply steady upwards and forward pressure to lift the mandible.

- Using the thumbs, slightly open the mouth by downward displacement of the chin.

These simple positional methods are successful in most cases where airway obstruction is caused by loss of muscle tone in the pharynx. After each manoeuvre, check for success using the look, listen and feel sequence. If a clear airway cannot be achieved, look for other causes of airway obstruction. Use a finger sweep to remove any solid foreign body visible in the mouth. Remove broken or displaced dentures but leave well-fitting dentures in place as they help to maintain the contours of the mouth, facilitating a good seal for ventilation by the mouth-to-mouth, mouth-to-mask or bag-mask techniques.

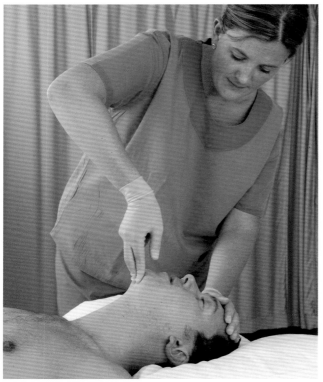

**Figure 6.1 Head tilt and chin lift**

## Jaw thrust

Jaw thrust is an alternative manoeuvre for bringing the mandible forward and relieving obstruction by the tongue (Figure 6.2). It is most successful when applied with a head tilt.

**ALS**

## Airway manoeuvres in a patient with suspected cervical spine injury

If spinal injury is suspected (e.g., if the victim has fallen, been struck on the head or neck, or has been rescued after diving into shallow water) maintain the head, neck, chest, and lumbar region in the neutral position during resuscitation. Excessive head tilt could aggravate the injury and damage the cervical spinal cord; however, this complication remains theoretical and the relative risk is unknown. When there is a risk of cervical spine injury, establish a clear upper airway by using jaw thrust or chin lift in combination with manual in-line stabilisation (MILS) of the head and neck by an assistant. If life-threatening airway obstruction persists despite effective application of jaw thrust or chin lift, add head tilt a small amount at a time until the airway is open; establishing a patent airway takes priority over concerns about a potential cervical spine injury.

# Adjuncts to basic airway techniques

Simple airway adjuncts are often helpful, and sometimes essential to maintain an open airway, particularly when resuscitation is prolonged. The position of the head and neck must be maintained to keep the airway aligned. Oropharyngeal and nasopharyngeal airways are designed to overcome soft palate obstruction and backward tongue displacement in an unconscious patient, but head tilt and jaw thrust may also be required.

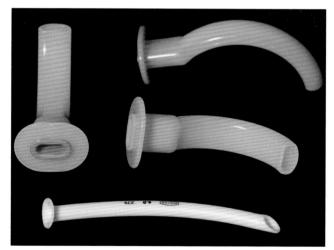

**Figure 6.3 Oropharyngeal and nasopharyngeal airways**

## Oropharyngeal airway

The oropharyngeal or Guedel airway is a curved plastic tube, flanged and reinforced at the oral end with a flattened shape to ensure that it fits neatly between the tongue and hard palate (Figure 6.3). It is available in sizes suitable for the new born to large adults. An estimate of the size required may be obtained by selecting an airway with a length corresponding to the vertical distance between the patient's incisors and the angle of the jaw (Figure 6.4). The most common sizes are 2, 3 and 4 for small, medium and large adults respectively.

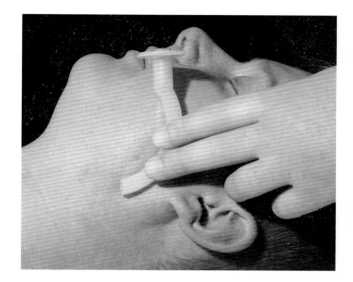

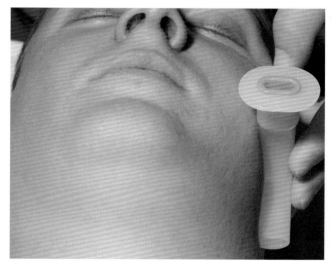

**Figure 6.4 Sizing of an oropharyngeal airway**

During insertion of an oropharyngeal airway, the tongue can occasionally be pushed backwards, exacerbating obstruction instead of relieving it. Ensuring a correct insertion technique should avoid this problem. Attempt insertion only in unconscious patients: vomiting or laryngospasm may occur if glossopharyngeal or laryngeal reflexes are present.

### Technique for insertion of oropharyngeal airway:

- Open the patient's mouth and ensure that there is no foreign material that may be pushed into the larynx (if there is any, then use suction to remove it).

- Insert the airway into the oral cavity in the 'upside-down' position as far as the junction between the hard and soft palate and then rotate it through 180° (Figure 6.5). Advance the airway until it lies in the pharynx. This rotation technique minimises the chance of pushing the tongue backwards and downwards. Remove the airway if the patient gags or strains. Correct placement is indicated by an improvement in airway patency and by the seating of the flattened reinforced section between the patient's teeth or gums (if edentulous).

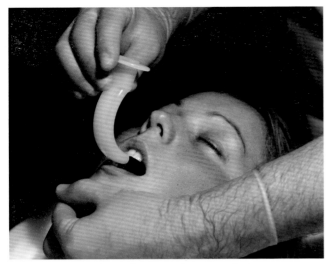

**Figure 6.5 Insertion of an oropharyngeal airway**

After insertion, maintain head tilt/chin lift or jaw thrust, and check the patency of the airway and ventilation using the look, listen and feel technique. Where there is suspicion of an injury to the cervical spine, maintain alignment and immobilisation of the head and neck. Suction is usually possible through an oropharyngeal airway using a fine bore flexible suction catheter.

## Nasopharyngeal airway

This is made from soft malleable plastic, bevelled at one end and with a flange at the other (Figure 6.3). In patients who are not deeply unconscious, it is better tolerated than an oropharyngeal airway. It may be life-saving in patients with clenched jaws, trismus or maxillofacial injuries.

Inadvertent insertion of a nasopharyngeal airway through a fracture of the skull base and into the cranial vault is possible, but extremely rare. In the presence of a known or suspected basal skull fracture an oral airway is preferred, but if this is not possible, and the airway is obstructed, gentle insertion of a nasopharyngeal airway may be life-saving (i.e., the benefits may far outweigh the risks).

The tubes are sized in millimetres according to their internal diameter, and the length increases with diameter. The traditional methods of sizing a nasopharyngeal airway (measurement against the patient's little finger or anterior nares) do not correlate with the airway anatomy and are unreliable. Sizes 6-7 mm are suitable for adults. Insertion can cause damage to the mucosal lining of the nasal airway, resulting in bleeding in up to 30% of cases. If the tube is too long it may stimulate the laryngeal or glossopharyngeal reflexes to produce laryngospasm or vomiting.

### Technique for insertion of nasopharyngeal airway

- Check for patency of the right nostril.

- Some designs require a safety pin to be inserted through the flange to provide an extra precaution against the airway disappearing beyond the nares.

- Lubricate the airway thoroughly using water-soluble jelly.

- Insert the airway bevel end first, vertically along the floor of the nose with a slight twisting action (Figure 6.6). The curve of the airway should direct it towards the patient's feet. If any obstruction is met, remove the tube and try the left nostril.

- Once in place, use the look, listen and feel technique to check the patency of the airway and adequacy of ventilation. Chin lift or jaw thrust may still be required to maintain airway patency. Where there is suspicion of an injury to the cervical spine, maintain correct alignment and immobilisation of the head and neck.

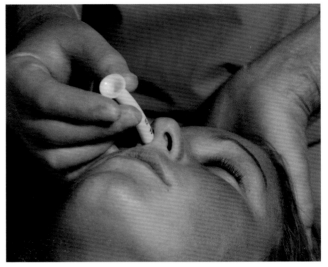

**Figure 6.6 Insertion of a nasopharyngeal airway**

## Oxygen

Always give oxygen when it is available. A venturi mask will deliver 24-60%, depending on the mask chosen. A standard oxygen mask will deliver up to 50%, providing the flow of oxygen is high enough. Initially, give the highest possible oxygen concentration—a mask with reservoir bag (non-rebreathing mask) can deliver an inspired oxygen concentration of 85% at flow rates of 10-15 l min⁻¹. Monitor the oxygen saturation by pulse oximeter ($SpO_2$) or arterial blood gases to enable titration of the inspired oxygen concentration.

## Suction

Use a wide bore rigid sucker (Yankauer) to remove liquid (blood, saliva and gastric contents) from the upper airway (Figure 6.7). Use the sucker cautiously if the patient has an intact gag reflex—it can provoke vomiting. Fine bore flexible suction catheters may be required in patients with limited mouth opening. These suction catheters can also be passed through oropharyngeal or nasopharyngeal airways.

ALS

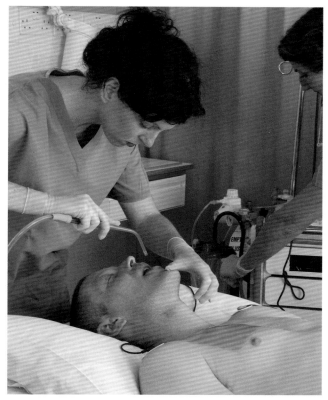

**Figure 6.7 Suction**

# Ventilation

Artificial ventilation is started as soon as possible in any patient in whom spontaneous ventilation is inadequate or absent. Expired air ventilation (rescue breathing) is effective but the rescuer's expired oxygen concentration is only 16-17%; so it must be replaced as soon as possible by ventilation with oxygen-enriched air. Although mouth-to-mouth ventilation has the benefit of not requiring any equipment, the technique is aesthetically unpleasant, particularly when vomit or blood is present, and the rescuer may be reluctant to place themselves in intimate contact with the victim who may be unknown to them.

There are only isolated reports of individuals acquiring infections after providing CPR, e.g., tuberculosis and severe acute respiratory distress syndrome (SARS). Transmission of HIV during provision of CPR has never been reported. Simple adjuncts are available to enable direct person-to-person contact to be avoided; some of these devices may reduce the risk of cross infection between patient and rescuer.

The pocket resuscitation mask is used widely. It is similar to an anaesthetic face mask and enables mouth-to-mask ventilation. It has a unidirectional valve, which directs the patient's expired air away from the rescuer. The mask is transparent so that vomit or blood from the patient can be seen. Some masks have a port for the addition of oxygen. When using masks without an oxygen port, supplemental oxygen can be given by placing oxygen tubing underneath one side and ensuring an adequate

seal. Use a two-hand technique to maximise the seal with the patient's face (Figure 6.8).

High airway pressures can be generated if the tidal volumes or inspiratory flows are too great, predisposing to gastric inflation and subsequent risk of regurgitation and pulmonary aspiration. As gastric inflation occurs lung compliance is further reduced making ventilation more difficult. The possibility of gastric inflation is increased by:

- Malalignment of the head and neck, and an obstructed airway.

- An incompetent oesophageal sphincter (present in all patients with cardiac arrest).

- A high inflation pressure.

Although relatively large tidal volumes (10 ml kg$^{-1}$) are necessary during expired-air ventilation, when supplemental oxygen is used, low tidal volumes in the region of 400-600 ml (6-7 ml kg$^{-1}$) will provide adequate oxygenation and ventilation, and will reduce the risk of gastric inflation. If inspiratory flow is too low, inspiratory time will be prolonged and the time available to give chest compressions is reduced. Deliver each breath over approximately one second and give a volume that corresponds to visible chest movement; this represents a compromise between giving an adequate volume, minimising the risk of gastric inflation, and allowing adequate time for chest compressions. During CPR with an unprotected airway, give two ventilations after each sequence of 30 chest compressions.

## Technique for mouth-to-mask ventilation

- Place the patient supine with the head in a 'sniffing' position i.e., neck slightly flexed on a pillow with the head extended (tilted backwards) on the neck.

- Apply the mask to the patient's face using the thumbs of both hands.

- Lift the jaw into the mask with the remaining fingers by exerting pressure behind the angles of the jaw (jaw thrust). At the same time, press the mask onto the face with the thumbs to make a tight seal (Figure 6.8).

- Blow through the inspiratory valve and watch the chest rise.

- Stop inflation and observe the chest falling.

- Any leaks between the face and mask can be reduced by adjusting the contact pressure, altering the position of the fingers and thumbs, or increasing jaw thrust.

- If oxygen is available, add it via the port at a flow of 10 l min$^{-1}$.

**ALS**

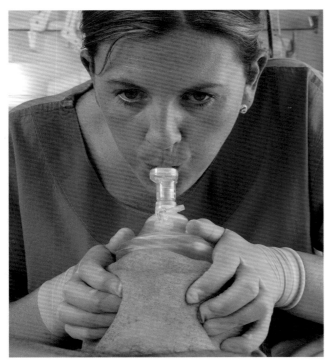

**Figure 6.8 Mouth-to-mask ventilation**

## Self-inflating bag

The self-inflating bag can be connected to a face mask, tracheal tube, or alternative airway devices such as the LMA or Combitube. As the bag is squeezed, the contents are delivered to the patient's lungs. On release, the expired gas is diverted to the atmosphere via a one-way valve; the bag then refills automatically via an inlet at the opposite end. When used without supplemental oxygen, the self-inflating bag ventilates the patient's lungs with only ambient air (oxygen concentration 21%). This is increased to around 45% by attaching an oxygen flow of 5-6 l min$^{-1}$ directly to the bag adjacent to the air intake. An inspired oxygen concentration of approximately 85% is achieved if a reservoir system is attached and the oxygen flow is increased to approximately 10 l min$^{-1}$. As the bag re-expands it fills with oxygen from both the reservoir and the continuous flow from the attached oxygen tubing.

Although the bag-mask apparatus enables ventilation with high concentrations of oxygen, its use by a single person requires considerable skill. When used with a face mask, it is often difficult to achieve a gas-tight seal between the mask and the patient's face, and maintain a patent airway with one hand whilst squeezing the bag with the other. Any significant leak will cause hypoventilation and if the airway is not patent, gas may also be forced into the stomach. This will reduce ventilation further and greatly increase the risk of regurgitation and aspiration. There is a natural tendency to try to compensate for a leak by excessive compression of the bag, which causes high peak airway pressures and forces more gas into the stomach. Some self-inflating bags have flow restrictors that limit peak airway pressure with the aim of reducing gastric inflation. Cricoid pressure can further reduce the risk of gastric inflation but requires the

presence of a trained assistant. Poorly applied cricoid pressure may make it more difficult to ventilate the patient's lungs.

The two-person technique for bag-mask ventilation is preferable (Figure 6.9). One person holds the face mask in place using a jaw thrust with both hands and an assistant squeezes the bag. In this way, a better seal can be achieved and the patient's lungs can be ventilated more effectively and safely.

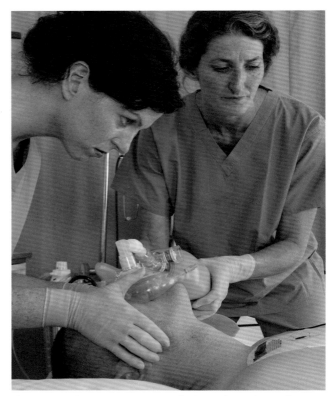

**Figure 6.9 The two-person technique for using a bag-mask ventilation**

## Key learning points

- Maintaining airway patency and ventilating the lungs are important components of CPR.

- Use of simple airway manoeuvres, with or without basic adjuncts, will often achieve a patent airway.

- Give all patients high concentration oxygen until the arterial oxygen saturation is known.

**ALS**

## Objectives

To understand:

▶ **The role of the LMA and other supraglottic airway devices during CPR.**

# Introduction

Effective bag-mask ventilation requires a reasonable level of skill and experience: the inexperienced are likely to achieve ineffective tidal volumes and cause gastric inflation with risk of regurgitation and pulmonary aspiration. In comparison with bag-mask ventilation, use of the laryngeal mask airway (LMA) and other supraglottic airway devices that sit above the larynx may enable more effective ventilation and reduce the risk of gastric inflation.

Without adequate training and experience, the incidence of complications associated with attempted tracheal intubation is unacceptably high. Unrecognised oesophageal intubation is disastrous and prolonged attempts at tracheal intubation are harmful: the cessation of chest compressions during this time will compromise coronary and cerebral perfusion. The alternative airway devices can be used if attempted intubation has failed or when personnel skilled in intubation are unavailable.

The LMA, the Combitube, and the Laryngeal Tube (LT) are the only alternative airway devices to be studied during CPR, but none of these studies has included enough subjects to enable their impact on survival to be determined. Most researchers have studied only insertion and ventilation success rates. There are no data supporting the routine use of any specific approach to airway management during cardiac arrest. The best technique is dependent on the precise circumstances of the cardiac arrest and the competence of the rescuer.

# Laryngeal mask airway (LMA)

The LMA consists of a wide bore tube with an elliptical inflated cuff designed to seal around the laryngeal opening (Figure 6.10). It was introduced into anaesthetic practice in the middle of the 1980s and has been shown to be a reliable and safe device, which can be introduced easily, with a high success rate after a short period of training. Ventilation using the LMA is more efficient and easier than with a bag-mask apparatus; provided high inflation pressures (>20 cm $H_2O$) are avoided, gastric inflation is minimised. When an LMA can be inserted without delay it is preferable to avoid bag-mask ventilation altogether: the risk of gastric inflation and regurgitation is reduced. Though not guaranteeing protection of the airway from gastric contents, pulmonary aspiration during use of the LMA is uncommon. The LMA does seem to protect against sources of aspiration from above the larynx. Furthermore, as the insertion of the LMA does not require extensive movement of the head and neck, it may be the airway device of choice in the presence of a suspected cervical spine injury. Use of the LMA by nursing, paramedical and medical staff during resuscitation has been studied and reported to be effective. Like tracheal intubation, it requires the patient to be deeply unconscious. The LMA is particularly valuable if attempted intubation by skilled personnel has failed and bag-mask ventilation is impossible (the cannot ventilate, cannot intubate scenario). The conventional LMA (LMA Classic™) can be reused up to 40 times after sterilisation. Single-use versions are now available and may be especially suitable for prehospital use. Some of the single-use LMAs are of a slightly different design and material to the LMA Classic™ and their performance may not be quite the same.

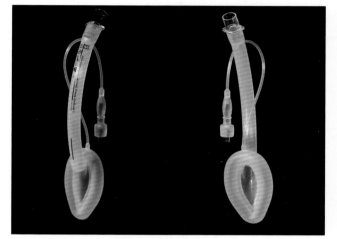

**Figure 6.10 Laryngeal mask airway**

### Technique for insertion of a laryngeal mask airway

- Select a LMA of an appropriate size for the patient and deflate the cuff fully. A size 5 will be correct for most men and a size 4 for most women. Lubricate the outer face of the cuff area (the part that will not be in contact with the larynx) with water-soluble gel.

- Flex the patient's neck slightly and extend the head (try to maintain neutral alignment of the head neck if there is suspicion of cervical spine injury).

- Holding the LMA like a pen, insert it into the mouth (Figure 6.11). Advance the tip behind the upper incisors with the upper surface applied to the palate until it reaches the posterior pharyngeal wall. Press the mask backwards and downwards around the corner of the pharynx until a resistance is felt as it locates in the back of the pharynx. If possible, get an assistant to apply a jaw thrust after the LMA has been inserted into the mouth - this increases the space in the posterior pharynx and makes successful placement easier.

- Connect the inflating syringe and inflate the cuff with air (40 ml for a size 5 LMA and 30 ml for a size 4 LMA); alternatively, inflate the cuff to a pressure of 60 cm $H_2O$. If insertion is satisfactory, the tube will lift 1-2 cm out of the mouth as the cuff finds its correct position and the larynx is pushed forward.

- If the LMA has not been inserted successfully after 30 sec, oxygenate the patient using a pocket mask or bag-mask before reattempting LMA insertion.

- Confirm a clear airway by listening over the chest during inflation and observing bilateral chest movement. A large, audible leak suggests malposition of the LMA, but a small leak is acceptable provided chest rise is adequate.

- Insert a bite block alongside the tube if available and secure the LMA with a bandage or tape.

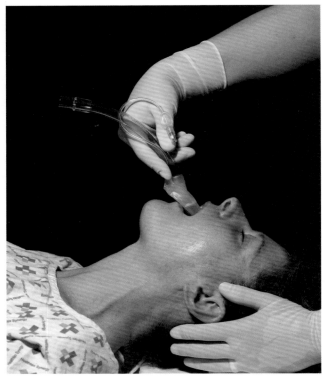

**Figure 6.11 Insertion of a laryngeal mask airway**

## Limitations of the LMA

- In the presence of high airway resistance or poor lung compliance (pulmonary oedema, bronchospasm, chronic obstructive pulmonary disease) there is a risk of a significant leak around the cuff causing hypoventilation. Most of the gas leaking around the cuff normally escapes through the patient's mouth but some gastric inflation may occur.

- There are no data demonstrating whether or not it is possible to provide adequate ventilation via an LMA without interruption of chest compressions. Uninterrupted chest compressions are likely to cause at least some gas leak from the LMA cuff when ventilation is attempted. Attempt continuous compressions initially but abandon this if persistent leaks and hypoventilation occur.

- There is a theoretical risk of aspiration of stomach contents because the LMA does not sit within the larynx like a tracheal tube; however, this complication has not been documented widely in clinical practice.

- If the patient is not deeply unconscious, insertion of the LMA may cause coughing, straining or laryngeal spasm. This will not occur in patients in cardiorespiratory arrest.

- If an adequate airway is not achieved, withdraw the LMA, deflate the cuff and attempt reinsertion ensuring a good alignment of the head and neck.

- Uncommonly, airway obstruction may be caused by the epiglottis folding down to cover the laryngeal inlet. Withdraw the LMA, deflate the cuff and attempt reinsertion.

To become proficient in the insertion of an LMA requires practice on patients and this should be achieved under the supervision of an appropriately experienced person (e.g., anaesthetist) in a controlled environment.

## The ProSeal LMA

The ProSeal LMA (PLMA) is a modified version of the original LMA. It has an additional posterior cuff and a gastric drain tube (Figure 6.12). The device has been studied extensively in anaesthetised patients, but there are no studies of its function and performance during CPR. It has several attributes that, in theory, make it more suitable than the original LMA for use during CPR: improved seal with the larynx enabling ventilation at higher airway pressures (commonly up to 35–40 cm $H_2O$), the inclusion of a gastric drain tube enabling venting of liquid regurgitated gastric contents from the upper oesophagus and passage of a gastric tube to drain liquid gastric contents, and the inclusion of a bite block. The higher seal pressures achieved with the PLMA may enable ventilation volume to be maintained during uninterrupted chest compressions. Potential weaknesses of the PLMA as an airway device for CPR are that it is slightly more difficult to insert than the original LMA, it is not available in disposable form at present, it is relatively expensive, and that solid regurgitated gastric contents could block the gastric drainage tube. Data are awaited on its performance during CPR.

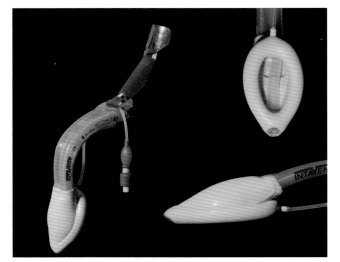

**Figure 6.12 ProSeal LMA**

# Other airway devices

## The Combitube

The Combitube is a double lumen tube introduced blindly over the tongue and into the pharynx (Figure 6.13). It is designed to provide a route for ventilation whether the tube has passed into the trachea or the oesophagus. The tracheal channel has an open distal end. The oesophageal tube has no terminal opening, but has several small side-holes located between two cuffs. There is a small distal cuff and a large proximal cuff designed to inflate within the pharynx.

When introduced blindly, the tube usually enters the oesophagus (in 95% of cases), and the patient's lungs are ventilated through the oesophageal channel via the side holes, which are located at or above the larynx (Figure 6.14a). Gas cannot pass down the oesophagus because of the blind end of the oesophageal channel, and the distal cuff, which is positioned just proximal to the blind end. The pharyngeal cuff prevents air leaking from the mouth. If the tube enters the trachea, ventilation is achieved via the tracheal port through its open distal end (Figure 6.14b).

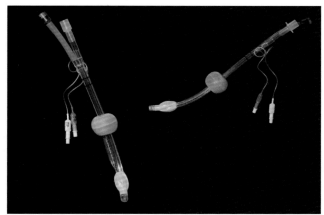

**Figure 6.13 The Combitube**

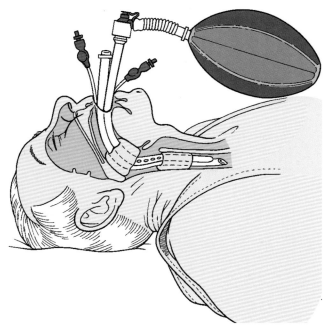

**Figure 6.14a Combitube in oesophageal position**

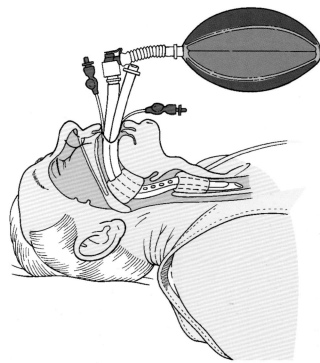

**Figure 6.14b Combitube in tracheal position**

### Limitations of the Combitube

- The device is relatively expensive.

- As with tracheal intubation and the LMA, adequate mouth opening is required and it may be impossible to insert if the patient's conscious level is not depressed sufficiently.

- Unlike the LMA, the Combitube cannot be inserted easily in the presence of a semi-rigid cervical collar.

- During insertion, sharp teeth can damage either of the cuffs.

- There have been reports of subcutaneous emphysema and oesophageal rupture associated with the Combitube. This may be because the device is relatively rigid and has a fixed anterior curve.

- In one retrospective review, the incorrect port was used for ventilation in 3.5% of cases. Ventilation of the wrong lumen will distend the stomach and this may lead to regurgitation and pulmonary aspiration.

ALS

## Laryngeal Tube

The Laryngeal Tube (LT) is one of many new supraglottic airway devices that have been developed. It is a single-lumen tube with both an oesophageal and pharyngeal cuff (Figure 6.15). A single pilot balloon inflates both cuffs simultaneously and it is available in a variety of sizes. Successful insertion and airway pressures generated are comparable to the LMA when performed by non-anaesthetists. There are sporadic case reports relating to use of the laryngeal tube during CPR and in one study, the LT was inserted by minimally trained nurses in 30 patients in cardiac arrest out of hospital.

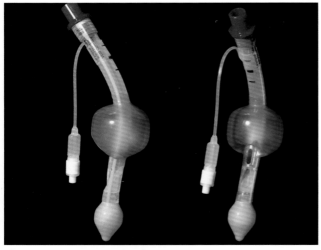

**Figure 6.15 Laryngeal Tube**

## Key learning points

- The LMA and Combitube are good alternatives to the bag-mask apparatus.

- These airway devices may be used instead of the tracheal tube whenever intubation has failed or is not possible because of lack of trained personnel.

- There are several new supraglottic airway devices. Few data are available to recommend their widespread use in the cardiopulmonary arrest setting at present.

### Objectives

To understand:

▶ **The advantages and disadvantages of tracheal intubation during cardiopulmonary resuscitation.**

▶ **Some simple aids to tracheal intubation.**

▶ **Some methods for confirming correct placement of a tracheal tube.**

▶ **The role of needle and surgical cricothyroidotomy.**

## Tracheal intubation

There is insufficient evidence to support or refute the use of any specific technique to maintain an airway and provide ventilation in adults with cardiorespiratory arrest. Despite this, tracheal intubation is perceived as the optimal method of providing and maintaining a clear and secure airway. It should be used only when trained personnel are available to carry out the procedure with a high level of skill and confidence. The only randomised controlled trial comparing tracheal intubation with bag-mask ventilation was undertaken in children requiring airway management out-of-hospital. In this study there was no difference in survival to discharge.

The perceived advantages of tracheal intubation over bag-mask ventilation include maintenance of a patent airway which is protected from aspiration of gastric contents or blood from the oropharynx, ability to provide an adequate tidal volume reliably even when chest compressions are uninterrupted, the potential to free the rescuers hands for other tasks, the ability to suction airway secretions and a potential route for giving drugs. Use of a bag-mask is more likely to cause gastric distension, which, theoretically, is more likely to cause regurgitation and the risk of aspiration. This theoretical risk has yet to be proven in randomised clinical trials.

The perceived disadvantages of tracheal intubation over bag-mask ventilation include the risk of an unrecognised misplaced tracheal tube (which is as high as 17% in some studies of out-of-hospital cardiac arrest), a prolonged time without chest compressions while tracheal intubation is attempted and a comparatively high failure rate. The cost of training prehospital staff to undertake intubation should also be considered. Healthcare personnel who undertake prehospital intubation should do so only within a structured, monitored program, which should include comprehensive competency-based training and regular opportunities to refresh skills.

In some cases, laryngoscopy and attempted intubation may

prove impossible or cause life-threatening deterioration in the patient's condition.* Such circumstances include acute epiglottitis, pharyngeal pathology, head injury (where coughing or straining may cause further increase in intracranial pressure), or in patients with cervical spine injury. In these circumstances, specialist skills such as the use of anaesthetic drugs or flexible fibreoptic laryngoscopy may be required. These techniques require a high level of skill and training.

Rescuers must weigh the risks and benefits of tracheal intubation against the need to provide effective chest compressions. The intubation attempt will require interruption of chest compressions but once an advanced airway is in place ventilation will not require any further interruption of chest compressions. Personnel skilled in advanced airway management should be able to undertake laryngoscopy without stopping chest compressions—a brief pause in chest compressions will be required as the tube is passed through the vocal cords. Alternatively, to avoid any interruptions in chest compressions, the intubation attempt may be deferred until return of spontaneous circulation. No intubation attempt should take longer than 30 sec: if intubation has not been achieved after this time, recommence bag-mask ventilation. After tracheal intubation, tube placement must be confirmed and the tube secured adequately. If there is any doubt about the correct position of the tube, remove it and reoxygenate the patient before making another attempt.

### Essential equipment for intubation

- Laryngoscope - generally a curved Macintosh blade. Several sizes are available, but a size 3 will be adequate for most patients. Check the light source and battery regularly and just before use, and ensure that spares are immediately available.

- Cuffed tracheal tubes - a selection should be available appropriate to the size of the patient. An 8.0 mm internal diameter tube is suitable for an adult male and a 7.0 mm internal diameter tube for a female.

- Sizes 6, 7 and 8 mm will generally cover the immediate needs of all adults. Availability of smaller tracheal tubes will be helpful for patients with conditions causing narrowing of the upper airway..

- Syringe for cuff inflation.

- Extras:

  - water-soluble lubricating jelly;

  - Magill's forceps;

  - introducers: either a gum elastic bougie or a semi-rigid stylet;

  - tape or bandage to secure tube in position;

  - stethoscope for confirming correct position of the tube;

  - suction apparatus with a wide-bore rigid suction end (e.g., Yankauer) and a range of smaller flexible catheters;

- exhaled $CO_2$ detection apparatus or oesophageal detector device to confirm correct tube placement. The oesophageal detector device is more reliable in cardiac arrest.

## Post-intubation procedures

- After successful intubation, connect the tracheal tube (via a catheter mount if necessary) to a ventilating device, e.g., self-inflating bag, and ventilate with the highest oxygen concentration available.

- Inflate the cuff of the tracheal tube just sufficiently to stop an air leak during inspiration.

- Listen over the epigastrium for evidence of gastric inflation. Observe chest movement and auscultate to check that both lungs are being ventilated. Listen at the sides of the chest (mid-axillary line) rather than anteriorly. If only the right side is being ventilated, it may indicate that the tube has been inserted too far, and has entered the right main bronchus: deflate the cuff, withdraw the tube 1-2 cm, reinflate the cuff and check ventilation. Use an exhaled $CO_2$ detector and/or oesophageal detector device to confirm correct tube placement (see below).

- Continue ventilation with a high concentration of oxygen.

- Secure the tube with a bandage or tie. Adhesive tape is not reliable if the face is moist.

- An oropharyngeal airway may be inserted alongside the tracheal tube to maintain the position of the tube, and prevent damage from biting when consciousness returns.

### Confirmation of correct tracheal tube placement

Confirmation of tracheal tube placement by an exhaled $CO_2$ or oesophageal detection device should reduce the risk of unrecognised oesophageal intubation. Neither of these techniques will differentiate a tube placed in a main bronchus from one placed correctly in the trachea.

The oesophageal detector device creates a suction force at the tracheal end of the tracheal tube, either from pulling back the plunger of a large syringe or releasing a compressed flexible bulb. Air is aspirated easily from the lower airways through a tracheal tube placed in the cartilage-supported rigid trachea. When the tube is in the oesophagus, air cannot be aspirated because the oesophagus collapses when aspiration is attempted. The oesophageal detector device is generally reliable in patients with both a perfusing and a non-perfusing rhythm but it may be misleading in patients with morbid obesity, late pregnancy, severe asthma or when there are copious tracheal secretions; in these conditions the trachea may collapse when aspiration is attempted.

Carbon dioxide detector devices measure the concentration of exhaled $CO_2$ from the lungs. The persistence of exhaled

$CO_2$ after six ventilations indicates placement of the tube in the trachea or a main bronchus. Confirmation of correct placement above the carina will require auscultation of the chest bilaterally in the mid-axillary lines. In patients with a spontaneous circulation, a lack of exhaled $CO_2$ indicates that the tube is in the oesophagus. During cardiac arrest, pulmonary blood flow may be so low that there is insufficient exhaled $CO_2$ for the detector to identify a correctly placed tracheal tube. When exhaled $CO_2$ is detected in cardiac arrest, it indicates reliably that the tube is in the trachea or main bronchus, but when it is absent, tracheal tube placement is best confirmed with an oesophageal detector device. A variety of electronic as well as simple, inexpensive, colorimetric $CO_2$ detectors are available for both in-hospital and out-of-hospital use.

## Potential problems during tracheal intubation

Anatomical and pathological variations that may make intubation difficult or impossible include receding lower jaw, short neck, prominent incisors, narrow mouth, stiff neck and trismus. If the vocal cords cannot be seen, do not attempt to insert the tube blindly. Often a gum-elastic bougie can be inserted through the glottis more easily than a tracheal tube and once in place the tube may be placed over the bougie and guided (rail-roaded) into the trachea. The intubating stylet may also be used to stiffen and pre-form the curvature of the tube or to guide it into the larynx. Problems during intubation may be caused by:

- Facial burns and trauma - it may be impossible to use BLS techniques or intubate patients with severe facial trauma or thermal injury to the upper airway. In such cases it may be necessary to establish a surgical airway, e.g., cricothyroidotomy.

- Upper airway pathology e.g., tumours, infection, swelling from anaphylaxis, etc.

- Insecure/loose teeth or dental prosthesis - these may be damaged or loosened if undue pressure is placed on them. Good intubation technique should reduce this risk.

- Gastric regurgitation - always have a functioning suction device and wide-bore suction to hand. Cricoid pressure may prevent passive regurgitation and pulmonary aspiration.

- Clenching of teeth - in the early stages of resuscitation good CPR may prevent the profound level of unconsciousness required for tracheal intubation. In this case, use basic airway and ventilation techniques.

- Oesophageal intubation – this should not go unrecognised if the recommended protocols are followed, particularly if tracheal tube placement is confirmed with an oesophageal detector device and/or capnometry. If in doubt, take the tube out and reoxygenate the lungs using a bag-mask.

- Possible cervical spine injury – suspect this in all patients who have a history of major blunt trauma. Use manual inline stabilisation (MILS) of the head and neck and ensure that intubation is undertaken by an experienced operator.

## Cricoid pressure

Cricoid pressure is applied to prevent regurgitation of gastric contents and the consequent risk of pulmonary aspiration. A trained assistant can carry it out during bag-mask ventilation and intubation. The cricoid cartilage is identified immediately below the thyroid cartilage where it forms a complete ring at the upper end of the trachea. A pressure of 30 N (3 kg) is applied anteroposteriorly, forcing the cricoid ring backwards to press the oesophagus against the vertebral column (Figure 6.16). Pressure is maintained until the tracheal tube is inserted through the vocal cords and the cuff has been inflated. The person carrying out the

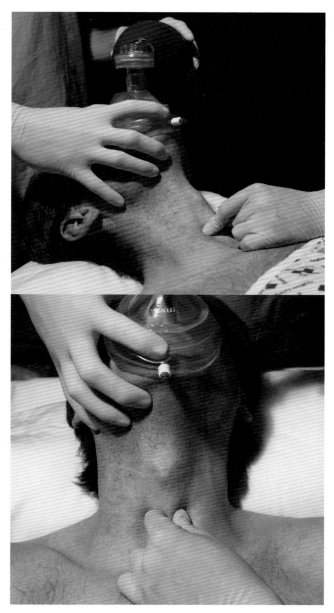

**Figure 6.16 Cricoid pressure**

intubation must indicate when pressure can be released. Do not apply cricoid pressure if there is active vomiting: it could cause oesophageal rupture. If cricoid pressure is applied imprecisely or with excessive force, ventilation with a bag-mask and tracheal intubation can be made more difficult. If ventilation of the patient's lungs is impossible, reduce the pressure applied to the cricoid cartilage or remove it completely.

## Aids to intubation

### Alternative laryngoscope blade

The Macintosh blade is a good general-purpose blade and a size 3 blade is suitable for most adults. Occasionally, a longer, size 4 blade is better for very large, long-necked patients. The McCoy levering laryngoscope has a hinged tip, and will often improve the view at laryngoscopy.

### Introducers

If visualisation is difficult, a gum-elastic bougie may be helpful to guide the tracheal tube into the larynx. It is best inserted into the larynx separately - the tube is then passed over it into the trachea. When correctly placed, free passage of the bougie is stopped by the smaller airways of the bronchial tree; a bougie placed accidentally in the oesophagus can be inserted completely, without obvious resistance. Ultimately, when ventilation and intubation are impossible and alternatives, e.g., an LMA, are not effective, it will be necessary to perform a cricothyroidotomy (see below).

Whilst descriptions of the advanced airway techniques above have been included, these descriptions are not intended as a substitute for practice on manikins, or on anaesthetised patients under the direction of an anaesthetist. Tracheal intubation during cardiac arrest should be attempted only by those undertaking the procedure regularly.

## Suction

Use a wide-bore rigid suction end (Yankauer) to remove liquid (blood, saliva and gastric contents) from the upper airway. This is done best under direct vision during intubation but must not delay achieving a definitive airway. Apply suction to the trachea as briefly as possible and ventilate the lungs with 100% oxygen before and after the procedure. Use fine-bore suction catheters for tracheal suction and pass them directly down the tracheal tube.

## Cricothyroidotomy

Occasionally it will be impossible to ventilate an apnoeic patient with a bag-mask, or to pass a tracheal tube or other airway device. This may occur in patients with extensive facial trauma or laryngeal obstruction caused by oedema, e.g., anaphylaxis, or foreign material. In these circumstances, it will be necessary to create a surgical airway below the level of the obstruction. A tracheostomy is contraindicated in an

ALS

emergency as it is time consuming, hazardous and requires considerable surgical skill and equipment. Substantial bleeding can occur. Needle or surgical cricothyroidotomy is the immediate technique of choice as it is less hazardous, more rapid, and requires only simple equipment.

## Needle cricothyroidotomy

### Procedure

- Place the patient supine with the head slightly extended.

- Identify the cricothyroid membrane as the recess between the thyroid cartilage and the cricoid cartilage.

- Puncture the membrane vertically in the midline using a large bore intravenous cannula or, preferably, a purpose-made cricothyroidotomy cannula, attached to a syringe (Figure 6.17). Aspiration of air confirms location in the trachea.

- Angle the cannula at 45° and advance caudally into the trachea. Remove the needle, confirm easy aspiration of air and attach the cannula to a high-pressure oxygen supply.

- Ventilate the patient's lungs by occluding the open limb of a Y connector or 3-way tap with a finger for one second, or until the chest rises adequately, then release for long enough to enable exhalation. Exhalation must occur through the larynx and upper airway. Do not attempt this technique if there is a total obstruction to exhalation by this route. If the larynx is partly occluded, allow adequate time for exhalation, otherwise the intrathoracic pressure will increase, reducing venous return and cardiac output, and causing pulmonary barotrauma.

- If a prepared Y connector or 3-way tap is not available, cut a hole in the oxygen supply tubing, and occlude intermittently with a finger to achieve ventilation.

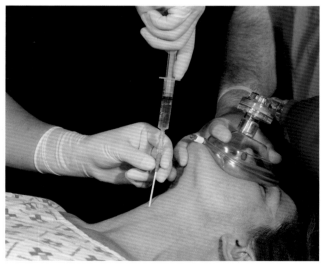

**Figure 6.17 Needle cricothyroidotomy**

Complications of needle cricothyroidotomy include insertion of the cannula outside the trachea causing massive surgical emphysema, haemorrhage, and oesophageal perforation.

## Surgical cricothyroidotomy

Unlike the needle cricothyroidotomy, the surgical technique will result in an airway that is protected by a cuffed tube. Higher airway pressures can be generated and tracheal suction is possible. Surgical cricothyroidotomy enables ventilation of the lungs despite complete airway obstruction at, or above, the glottis.

### Procedure for surgical cricothyroidotomy

- Place the patient supine with the head extended if possible.

- Identify the cricothyroid membrane as the recess just above the cricoid cartilage and below the thyroid cartilage.

- Incise the skin over the membrane and extend the incision through the cricothyroid membrane. Make a vertical incision in the skin and a horizontal one into the cricothyroid membrane; this avoids the superiorly positioned cricothyroid artery.

- Use the reversed handle of a scalpel or tissue expanding forceps to open up the incision in the cricothyroid membrane.

- Insert a suitably sized tracheal tube into the trachea and inflate the cuff. Do not insert the tube too far into the trachea: the carina is not far from here.

- Ventilate the lungs with a standard self-inflating bag attached to high flow oxygen. Exhalation occurs directly through the tracheal tube and tracheal suction is also now possible.

## Key learning points

- When undertaken by someone with appropriate skills and experience, tracheal intubation is the most effective airway management technique during cardiopulmonary resuscitation.

- In unskilled hands, prolonged interruptions of chest compressions, and the high risk of failure and other complications (e.g., unrecognised oesophageal intubation) make intubation attempts potentially harmful.

**ALS**

## Section 4. Basic mechanical ventilation

### Objectives

To understand:

▶ **The role of automatic ventilators in the peri-arrest period.**

There are very few studies that address specific aspects of ventilation during advanced life support. There are some data indicating that the ventilation rates delivered by healthcare personnel during cardiac arrest are excessive. Various small portable automatic ventilators may be used during resuscitation. They are usually gas powered. If an oxygen cylinder is used, both to supply the patient with oxygen and to power the ventilator, the contents may be used up rapidly. Most automatic resuscitators provide a constant flow of gas to the patient during inspiration; the volume delivered is dependent on the inspiratory time (a longer time provides a greater tidal volume). Because pressure in the airway rises during inspiration, these devices are often pressure-limited to protect the lungs against barotrauma. Expiration occurs passively into the atmosphere.

Set an automatic resuscitator initially to deliver a tidal volume of 6-7 ml kg$^{-1}$ at 10 breaths min$^{-1}$. Some ventilators have co-ordinated markings on the controls to facilitate easy and rapid adjustment for patients of different sizes, and others are capable of sophisticated variation in respiratory pattern. In the presence of a spontaneous circulation, the correct setting will be determined by checking the patient's arterial blood gas values. If a tracheal tube, LMA or Combitube has not been inserted, do not attempt chest compressions during the inspiratory phase. Once the patient has been intubated, or an LMA or Combitube inserted, it is unnecessary to interrupt chest compressions during inspiration.

Automatic resuscitators provide some advantages over alternative methods of ventilation:

- In intubated patients they free the rescuer for other tasks.

- In unintubated patients the rescuer has both hands free for mask and airway alignment.

- They provide a specific respiratory rate.

- If the patient is intubated, they provide a specific, relatively constant tidal volume.

Certain professional first responders (e.g., police, fire, and sports rescue personnel) may use simple automatic resuscitators provided that they have been trained adequately.

### Key learning points

- Automatic resuscitators may be a useful adjunct during cardiopulmonary resuscitation, although there are limited data on their use. Their safe use requires appropriate training.

## Further reading

Nolan JP, Deakin CD, Soar J, Bottiger BW, Smith G. European Resuscitation Council Guidelines for Resuscitation 2005. Section 4: Adult advanced life support. Resuscitation 2005;67 Suppl 1:S39-86.

International Liaison Committee on Resuscitation. Part 4. Advanced Life Support. 2005 International Consensus on Cardiopulmonary Resuscitation and Emergency Cardiovascular Care Science with Treatment Recommendations. Resuscitation 2005;67:213-247.

ALS

ALS

# Cardiac Monitoring, Electrocardiography, and Rhythm Recognition

## Objectives

To understand:

▶ **The reasons for ECG monitoring.**

▶ **How to monitor the ECG.**

▶ **The origin of the ECG.**

▶ **The importance of recording the ECG.**

▶ **The cardiac rhythms associated with cardiac arrest.**

▶ **How to identify other common arrhythmias.**

## Introduction

During cardiac arrest, identification of the cardiac rhythm will help to determine the correct treatment. Establish cardiac monitoring as soon as possible during cardiac arrest.

Some patients are at risk of developing an arrhythmia that may lead to cardiac arrest or other serious deterioration in their condition. Early detection and treatment of the arrhythmia may prevent cardiac arrest in some patients and prevent life-threatening deterioration in others. Patients at risk include those with chest pain, reduced conscious level, heart failure, palpitation, or shock. Establish cardiac monitoring in all patients at risk of serious arrhythmia.

When an arrhythmia occurs, single-lead monitoring may draw attention to it but may not always enable accurate rhythm recognition; whenever possible, record a 12-lead ECG to document the arrhythmia.

Single-lead ECG monitoring is not a reliable technique for detecting evidence of myocardial ischaemia (ST segment depression). Record serial 12-lead ECGs in patients experiencing chest pain suggestive of an acute coronary syndrome.

During cardiac arrest, recognition of ventricular fibrillation (VF) and pulseless ventricular tachycardia (VT) as shockable rhythms is crucial to the delivery of effective treatment. Automated external defibrillators (AEDs) and shock advisory defibrillators (SADs) can identify these rhythms reliably by electronic analysis. If a shockable rhythm is present, the defibrillator will charge to the appropriate energy level and instruct the operator that a shock is required. The introduction of AEDs has enabled resuscitation from VF/VT to be achieved by people who do not have skill in rhythm recognition, both in hospitals and in the community.

The accurate analysis of some cardiac rhythm abnormalities requires experience and expertise; however, the non-expert can interpret most rhythms sufficiently to identify the appropriate treatment. The main priority is to recognise that the rhythm is abnormal and that the heart rate is inappropriately slow or fast. Use the structured approach to rhythm interpretation in this chapter to avoid errors. The need for immediate treatment will be determined largely by the effect of the arrhythmia on the patient rather than by the nature of the arrhythmia. When an arrhythmia is present, first assess the patient, and then interpret the rhythm as accurately as possible. Treat the patient, not the ECG!

## Techniques for ECG monitoring

### Cardiac Monitors

Cardiac monitors display the ECG on a screen in real time. The signal is obtained from adhesive electrodes on the patient's skin and transmitted to the monitor either by wires or by telemetry. Many monitor systems have other features, such as the ability to print samples of the ECG rhythm display or to store samples of the ECG. Most modern monitors include a display of heart rate, and some have alarms that can be programmed to provide an alert when the heart rate goes below or exceeds preset limits. Many systems enable monitoring of other values such as blood pressure and oxygen saturation, which are important in the assessment of patients at risk. Digital processing of the ECG offers the potential for electronic analysis of the cardiac rhythm. If a patient requires monitoring, make sure that the monitor is being observed so that immediate action can be taken if necessary, should the rhythm change.

#### How to attach the monitor

Attach ECG electrodes to the patient using the positions shown in Figure 7.1. These will enable monitoring using 'modified limb leads' I, II or III. Make sure that the skin is dry, not greasy (use an alcohol swab and/or abrasive pad to clean), and either place the electrodes on relatively hair-free skin or shave off dense hair. Place electrodes over bone rather than muscle, to minimise interference from muscle artefact in the ECG signal. Different positions may be used when necessary (e.g., trauma, recent surgery, skin disease).

Many leads are colour-coded to help with correct connection. The usual scheme (except in the United States) uses **R**ed for the **R**ight arm lead, ye**LL**ow for the **L**eft arm lead, **G**reen for the le**G** lead (usually placed on the abdomen or lower left chest wall) for modified limb leads.

Begin by monitoring in modified lead II as this usually displays good amplitude sinus P waves and good amplitude QRS complexes, but switch to another lead if necessary to obtain the best ECG signal. Try to minimise muscle and movement artefact by explaining to patients what the monitoring is for and by keeping them warm and relaxed.

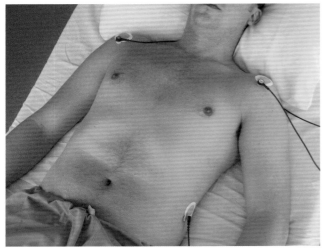

**Figure 7.1 Position of adhesive electrodes for monitoring the ECG using modified limb leads**

## Emergency monitoring

In an emergency, such as a collapsed patient, assess the cardiac rhythm as soon as possible. There are two options:

**Self-adhesive electrodes (pads)** can be used for monitoring and hands free shock delivery (Figure 7.2). Apply the electrodes in the conventional paddle positions, beneath the right clavicle and on the left chest wall. Use anterior and posterior positions as an alternative if the conventional positions cannot be used (e.g., permanent pacemaker in right pectoral position, left chest wall trauma).

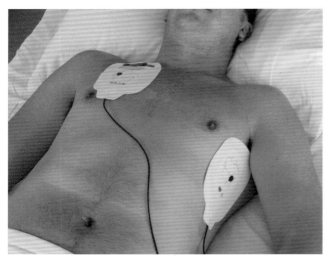

**Figure 7.2 Self-adhesive electrodes**

**Quick-look paddles.** Most manual defibrillators enable the ECG to be monitored through the paddles when they are applied to the chest wall (Figure 7.3). This is suitable only for a 'quick look' at cardiac rhythm. Do not interrupt chest compression for more than a few seconds to assess rhythm. When monitoring through paddles keep these very still to avoid movement artefact. Establish monitoring using adhesive electrodes and leads at the earliest possible time.

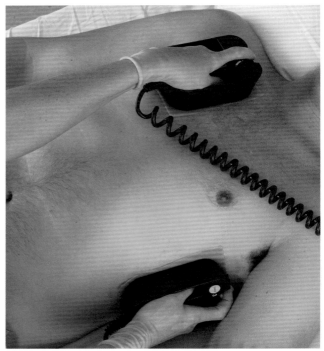

**Figure 7.3 Monitoring with paddles**

## Diagnosis from cardiac monitors

Use the displays and printouts from cardiac monitors only for rhythm recognition; do not attempt to interpret ST segment abnormalities or other more sophisticated elements of the ECG from monitors. When an arrhythmia is detected on a monitor, record a rhythm strip whenever possible.

If the arrhythmia persists for long enough, record a 12-lead ECG. It is not always possible to identify an arrhythmia from a single lead ECG recording. The heart is a three-dimensional organ and the 12-lead ECG examines the electrical signals from the heart in three dimensions. Sometimes, features that enable precise identification of cardiac rhythm are visible in only one or two leads of the 12-lead ECG and would not be seen on a single-lead recording of any other lead (Figure 7.4).

These recordings may assist with rhythm interpretation at the time but are also useful for later examination and planning of treatment in the longer term. Therefore effective management of any arrhythmia, including a cardiac arrest arrhythmia, includes good quality recording, as well as interpretation and treatment at the time.

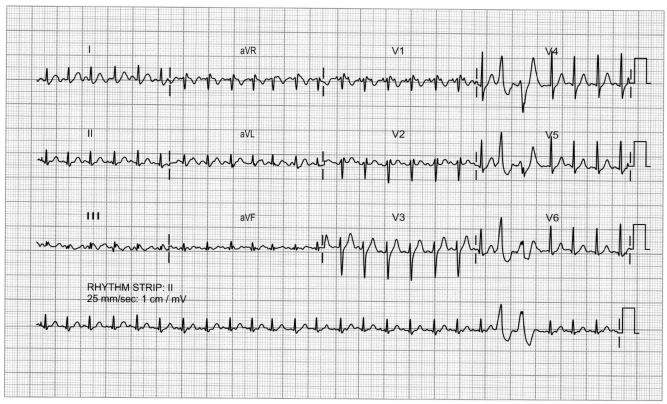

**Figure 7.4 12-lead ECG - atrial tachycardia seen clearly only in lead V1**

Adenosine given

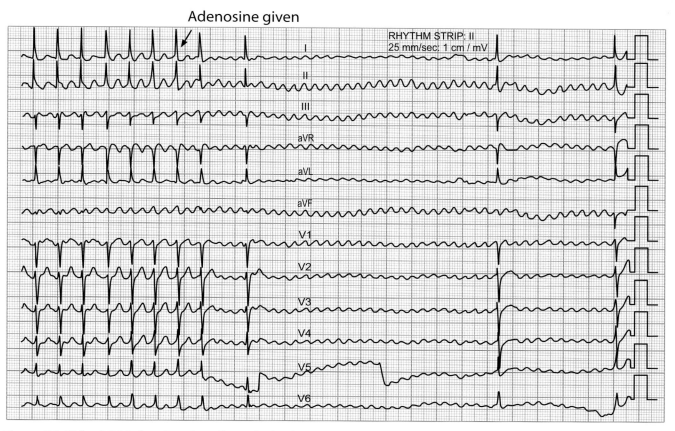

**Figure 7.5 12-lead ECG showing the effect of adenosine in atrial flutter. Transient AV block demonstrates clearly that this regular narrow-complex tachycardia was atrial flutter with 2:1 AV conduction.**

Valuable information about the nature and origin of a tachyarrhythmia can also be obtained by recording the response to treatment (e.g., carotid sinus massage, adenosine). Whenever possible, the effect of any such intervention should be recorded on a continuous ECG print-out, if possible using multiple leads (Figure 7.5).

# Basic Electrocardiography

At rest, the cells of the cardiac conducting system and myocardium are polarised. A potential difference of approximately 90 mV is present between the inside of the cell (which is negatively charged) and the extracellular space. A sudden shift of calcium and/or sodium ions across the cell membrane triggers depolarisation, generating the electrical signal that travels through the conducting system and triggers contraction of myocardial cells.

In normal sinus rhythm, depolarisation begins in a group of specialised 'pacemaker' cells, called the sino-atrial (SA) node, located close to the entry of the superior vena cava into the right atrium. A wave of depolarisation then spreads from the SA node through the atrial myocardium. This is seen on the ECG as the P wave (Figure 7.6). Atrial contraction is the mechanical response to this electrical impulse.

The transmission of this electrical impulse to the ventricles occurs through specialised conducting tissue (Figure 7.7).

Firstly, there is slow conduction through the atrioventricular (AV) node, followed by rapid conduction to the ventricular myocardium by specialised conducting tissue (Purkinje fibres). The bundle of His carries these fibres from the AV node and then divides into right and left bundle branches, spreading out through the right and left ventricles respectively. Rapid conduction down these fibres ensures that the ventricles contract in a co-ordinated fashion.

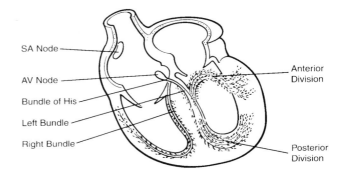

**Figure 7.7 Electrical conduction in the heart**

Depolarisation of the bundle of His, bundle branches and ventricular myocardium is seen on the ECG as the QRS complex (Figure 7.6). Ventricular contraction is the mechanical response to this electrical impulse.

Between the P wave and QRS complex is a small isoelectric segment, which largely represents the delay in transmission through the AV node. The normal sequence of atrial depolarisation followed by ventricular depolarisation (P wave followed by QRS complex) is sinus rhythm (Rhythm Strip 1).

The T wave, which follows the QRS complex, represents recovery of the resting potential in the cells of the conducting system and ventricular myocardium (ventricular repolarisation).

Because the normal conducting system transmits the depolarising impulse rapidly to both ventricles, the normal QRS complex is of relatively short duration (normally less than 0.12 sec).

When one of the bundle branches is diseased or damaged, rapid conduction to the corresponding ventricle is prevented. The depolarising impulse travels more rapidly down the other bundle branch to its ventricle and then more slowly, through ordinary ventricular myocardium to the other ventricle. This situation is called bundle branch block. Because depolarisation of both ventricles takes longer than normal it is seen on the ECG as a broad QRS complex (0.12 sec or longer).

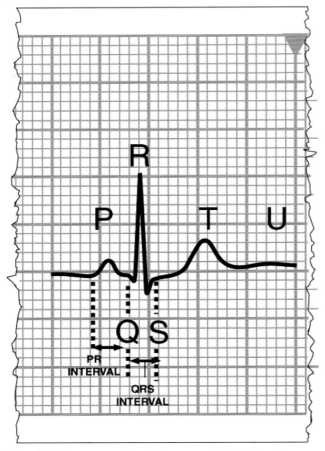

**Figure 7.6 Components of the normal ECG signal**

ALS

# How to read a rhythm strip

Experience and expertise may be needed to identify some rhythm abnormalities with complete precision. However, a simple, structured approach to interpreting the rhythm on any ECG recording will define any rhythm in sufficient detail to enable the most appropriate treatment to be chosen.

Apply the following 6-stage system to the analysis of any rhythm on an ECG:

1. Is there any electrical activity?

2. What is the ventricular (QRS) rate?

3. Is the QRS rhythm regular or irregular?

4. Is the QRS complex width normal or prolonged?

5. Is atrial activity present?

6. Is atrial activity related to ventricular activity and, if so, how?

Any cardiac rhythm can be described accurately (e.g., irregular narrow complex tachycardia, regular broad-complex bradycardia, etc.) and managed safely and effectively using the first four steps.

## Is there any electrical activity?

If you cannot see any electrical activity, check that the gain control is not too low and that the electrodes and leads are connected to both the patient and the monitor.

Check the patient: is a pulse present? If the patient is pulseless and there is still no activity on the ECG this is asystole (Rhythm Strip 2). Atrial and ventricular asystole are often both present, resulting in a line with no deflections. A completely straight line indicates usually that a monitoring lead has become disconnected. During asystole the ECG usually shows slight undulation of the baseline, and may show electrical interference due to respiratory movement, or chest compression.

Atrial activity (usually P waves but occasionally atrial fibrillation (AF) or atrial flutter) may continue for a short time after the onset of ventricular asystole. The ECG will show the atrial activity but no QRS complexes – ventricular standstill (Rhythm Strip 3). Recognition of this is important because pacing is more likely to achieve a cardiac output in this situation than in most cases of complete asystole (Chapter 11).

If the patient is pulseless and electrical activity is present, decide whether recognisable QRS complexes are present. If not, and the ECG shows rapid, bizarre, irregular deflections of random frequency and amplitude, this is ventricular fibrillation (Rhythm Strip 4). In ventricular fibrillation (VF) all co-ordination of electrical activity is lost, and there is no effective ventricular contraction, and no detectable cardiac output.

Ventricular fibrillation is sometimes classified as coarse (Rhythm Strip 4) or fine (Rhythm Strip 5) depending on the amplitude of the complexes; If there is doubt about whether the rhythm is asystole or fine VF, do not attempt defibrillation; instead, continue chest compressions and ventilation. Fine VF that is difficult to distinguish from asystole is unlikely to be shocked successfully into a perfusing rhythm. Continuing good quality CPR may improve the amplitude and frequency of the VF and improve the chance of subsequent successful defibrillation to a perfusing rhythm. Delivering repeated shocks in an attempt to defibrillate what is thought to be fine VF will increase myocardial injury both directly from the electric current and indirectly from the interruptions in coronary blood flow (Chapter 5).

If electrical activity is present and contains recognisable QRS complexes, continue with the following steps in rhythm analysis.

If the patient is pulseless and there are recognisable complexes on the ECG that would be expected to produce a pulse, this is pulseless electrical activity (PEA) and requires immediate CPR. Do **not** delay CPR whilst the rhythm is analysed.

## What is the ventricular (QRS) rate?

The normal heart rate (ventricular rate) at rest is 60-100 beats min$^{-1}$. A bradycardia has a heart rate slower than 60 min$^{-1}$. A tachycardia has a rate faster than 100 min$^{-1}$. ECG paper is calibrated in mm, with bolder lines every 5 mm. Standard paper speed is 25 mm sec$^{-1}$. One second is represented by 5 large squares (25 small squares).

One quick method for estimating the ventricular rate is to count the number of large (5 mm) squares between two consecutive QRS complexes and divide this number into 300 (e.g., in Rhythm Strip 1 there are 4 large squares between adjacent QRS complexes so the rate is 300/4 = 75 min$^{-1}$). This is less useful in irregular rhythms because the intervals between QRS complexes are not constant.

It is not accurate when the interval between QRS complexes does not correspond to an exact number of large squares. In this situation count the number of small squares between adjacent QRS complexes and divide into 1500 (e.g., in Rhythm Strip 1 there are 20 small squares between adjacent QRS complexes, so the rate is 1500/20 = 75 min$^{-1}$).

Alternatively, count the number of cardiac cycles in a defined number of seconds and calculate the rate per minute. For example, if 8 cardiac cycles occur in 30 large squares (6 sec), or 4 cycles in 15 large squares (3 sec) the rate is 80 min$^{-1}$ (Figure 7.8).

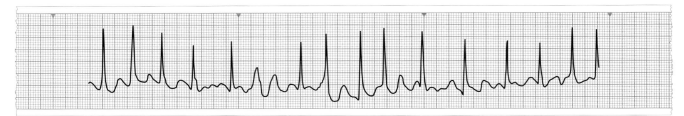

**Figure 7.8 Calculation of heart rate from a rhythm strip. (8 cardiac cycles occur in 30 large squares = 80 min⁻¹)**

## Is the QRS rhythm regular or irregular?

This is not always as easy as it seems; at faster heart rates beat-to-beat variation during some irregular rhythms appears less obvious. Some rhythms may be regular in places but intermittent variation in R-R interval makes them irregular.

Inspect an adequate length of rhythm strip carefully, measuring out each R-R interval and comparing it to others to detect any irregularity that is not obvious at first glance. Callipers or dividers are very useful for comparing the R-R intervals. Alternatively, the position of two adjacent identical points in the cardiac cycle (such as the tips of the R waves) can be marked on a strip of paper; this can then be moved to another section of the rhythm strip. If the rhythm is regular the marks will align precisely with each pair of R waves.

If the QRS rhythm is irregular, decide:

- Is this totally irregular, with no recognisable pattern of R-R interval?

- Is the basic rhythm regular, with intermittent irregularity?

- Is there a recurring cyclical variation in the R-R intervals?

If there is a cyclical pattern, the relationship between the QRS waves and the P wave requires careful analysis, as described below. If the R-R intervals are totally irregular (irregularly irregular) and the QRS complex is of constant morphology, the rhythm is most likely to be atrial fibrillation (Rhythm Strip 6).

A regular underlying rhythm may be made irregular by extrasystoles (ectopic beats). Extrasystoles can arise from the atria or the ventricles, and the position or focus from which they arise will determine their morphology on an ECG.

If the QRS complex of ectopic beats is narrow (< 0.12 sec), the beat is likely to have come from above the ventricular myocardium (i.e., from atrial muscle or the AV node).

Broad-complex ectopic beats may be of ventricular origin or may be supraventricular ectopic beats with bundle branch block.

Broad-complex atrial premature beats can sometimes be identified by a preceding ectopic P wave. Ventricular ectopic beats can be accompanied by a P wave occurring shortly after the QRS complex, caused by retrograde conduction from the ventricles to the atria.

Ectopic beats that occur early (that is before the next regular sinus beat was due to occur) are referred to as premature beats (Rhythm Strip 7).

A beat that arises from the AV node or from ventricular myocardium after a long pause, for example during sinus bradycardia or after sinus arrest, is referred to as an escape beat (Rhythm Strip 8). This implies that the focus in the AV node or ventricle that generates this beat is acting as a back-up pacemaker, because the normal pacemaker function of the sinus node is too slow or absent. Ectopic beats may occur singly, in pairs (couplets) or in threes (triplets). If more than three ectopic beats occur in rapid succession, this is regarded as a tachyarrhythmia.

An arrhythmia that occurs intermittently, interspersed with periods of normal sinus rhythm, is described as paroxysmal.

When ectopic beats occur alternately with sinus beats for a sustained period this is called bigeminy. It may be referred to as atrial bigeminy or ventricular bigeminy, depending on whether the ectopic beats are atrial or ventricular in origin.

## Is the QRS complex width normal or prolonged?

The upper limit of normal for the QRS interval is 0.12 sec (3 small squares). If the QRS width is less than this, the rhythm originates from above the bifurcation of the bundle of His and may be from the SA node, atria or AV node, but not from the ventricular myocardium. If the QRS duration is 0.12 sec or more the rhythm may be coming from ventricular myocardium or may be a supraventricular rhythm, transmitted with aberrant conduction (i.e., bundle branch block).

## Is atrial activity present?

Having defined the rhythm in terms of rate, regularity and QRS width, examine the ECG carefully for evidence of atrial activity. This may be difficult or impossible to identify, either because it is not visible or because atrial activity is partly or completely obscured by QRS complexes or T waves. Do not guess or try to convince yourself that you can identify atrial activity unless you are completely sure.

**ALS**

Depending on the nature of the arrhythmia and the ECG lead being examined, P waves may be present as positive deflections, negative deflections or biphasic deflections. When present, U waves may be mistaken for P waves. P waves may coincide with and cause distortion or variation of QRS complexes, ST segments, or T waves. Whenever possible, recording of a 12-lead ECG may enable P waves to be identified in one or more leads, even if they cannot be seen clearly in the initial monitoring lead. Lead V1 is often useful for clear demonstration of some types of atrial activity including sinus P waves and atrial fibrillation. Sinus P waves are usually seen clearly in lead II.

Other types of atrial activity may be present. During atrial flutter, atrial activity is seen as flutter waves - an absolutely regular repetitive deflection with a 'saw-tooth' appearance, often at a rate of about 300 min-1. This is usually seen best in the inferior leads (II, III, aVF) (Figure 7.5).

During AF, circuits and waves of depolarisation travel randomly through both atria. There are no P waves. Atrial fibrillation waves may be seen as rapid deviations from the baseline of varying amplitude and duration, usually seen best in lead V1. In some patients this may be of such low amplitude that no atrial activity can be seen.

During a sustained tachycardia atrial activity may not be visible. If the rhythm is of atrial origin (e.g. atrial flutter or AF) it may be possible to reveal atrial activity by slowing the ventricular rate whilst recording an ECG, preferably in multiple leads. For example, if a regular tachycardia of 150 min-1 is due to atrial flutter with 2:1 block it may not be possible to identify flutter waves with confidence. A transient increase in AV block by vagal stimulation or by an intravenous bolus of adenosine will demonstrate the flutter waves and identify the rhythm accurately (Figure 7.5).

The shape and direction of P waves help to identify the atrial rhythm. For example, sinus P waves are upright in leads II and aVF. If retrograde activation of the atria is taking place from the region of the AV node (i.e., the rhythm is junctional or ventricular in origin), the P waves will be inverted in leads II and aVF because atrial depolarisation travels in the opposite direction to normal.

P wave rate and regularity (and flutter wave rate) are assessed in the same way as the rate and regularity of QRS complexes.

### Is atrial activity related to ventricular activity and, if so, how?

If there is a consistent interval between each P wave and the following QRS complex, it is likely that conduction between atrium and ventricle is intact and that ventricular depolarisation is triggered by atrial depolarisation. Examine a long rhythm strip to make sure that subtle variation in the PR interval is not missed. Occasionally conduction between atria and ventricles is reversed (i.e., ventricular depolarisation is followed by retrograde conduction through the AV node and then by atrial depolarisation); the P wave occurs soon

after the QRS complex. It may sometimes be difficult to distinguish between this situation and the presence of a very long PR interval.

In other circumstances careful inspection will detect no relationship between the timing of P waves and of QRS complexes. This will indicate that atrial and ventricular depolarisation is arising independently, referred to as atrioventricular dissociation. Examples of this include:

- Complete (third degree) AV block, where a normal sinus rate in the atria is accompanied by a regular bradycardia arising below the AV node.

- Some examples of VT in which regular broad QRS complexes are present and regular P waves can be seen at a different, slower rate, out of phase with the QRS complexes.

Difficulty may arise when the relationship between the P waves and the QRS complexes varies in a recurring pattern. This may be misinterpreted as atrioventricular dissociation. This is seen most commonly in one form of second degree AV block (called Wenkebach or Mobitz I AV block). Examine a long rhythm strip carefully for recurring patterns and plot and compare the timing of P waves and QRS complexes. In complete AV block, the QRS rhythm is usually completely regular.

In AF, the atrial activity is completely irregular, so there is no identifiable relationship between this atrial activity and the irregular ventricular rhythm that results from it. If AF is accompanied by a completely regular, slow ventricular rhythm this is likely to be due to complete AV block in the presence of AF in the atria.

In atrial flutter there may be a consistent relationship between the flutter waves and the QRS complexes, giving rise to 1:1, 2:1, 3:1 conduction etc. In some instances, there is a constantly varying relationship, producing an irregular QRS rhythm; this is atrial flutter with variable AV block.

## Cardiac arrest rhythms

The rhythms present during cardiac arrest can be classified into 3 groups:

- ventricular fibrillation (VF) and some cases of ventricular tachycardia (VT);

- asystole;

- pulseless electrical activity (PEA).

Extreme bradycardia and rarely very fast supraventricular tachyarrhythmia may also cause such a severe fall in cardiac output to effectively cause cardiac arrest.

### Ventricular fibrillation

The characteristic appearance of VF (Rhythm Strip 4) is usually easy to recognise, and this is the only rhythm that does not need the systematic rhythm analysis described earlier in this chapter. When a monitor appears to show VF check the patient immediately to establish whether this is VF requiring immediate defibrillation, or whether the appearance is due to artefact. If the patient has a pulse, the rhythm is not VF.

Two rhythm abnormalities may resemble VF in some circumstances, since both produce an irregular, broad-complex, fast rhythm:

One is polymorphic VT. This may cause cardiac arrest, and when it does so the immediate treatment is the same as for VF, so failure to distinguish this immediately from VF would not lead to inappropriate treatment. However, it is important to document polymorphic VT and to recognise it following immediate resuscitation, so that the causes can be identified and corrected and appropriate treatment given to prevent recurrence.

The second possible source of confusion is AF in the presence of an accessory pathway connecting atrial and ventricular muscle (Wolff-Parkinson-White (WPW) syndrome). Some of these accessory pathways can conduct very rapidly, transmitting atrial impulses to the ventricles, sometimes at 300 min$^{-1}$ or faster. This produces an irregular broad complex tachycardia (Figure 7.9) that might be mistaken for VF or polymorphic VT. Left untreated, this rhythm may lead to VT or VF causing cardiac arrest. If AF with WPW syndrome itself caused clinical cardiac arrest, the correct treatment would be immediate defibrillation (as for any broad-complex pulseless tachycardia) so, again,

misinterpretation as VF or VT would not lead to inappropriate treatment. Again, the importance of documenting and recognising the rhythm is to ensure that the patient receives immediate appropriate specialist referral for treatment to protect them against the risk of recurrence of this potentially dangerous arrhythmia.

## Ventricular tachycardia

Ventricular tachycardia (VT) may cause loss of cardiac output resulting in cardiac arrest, particularly at faster rates or in the presence of structural heart disease (e.g., impaired left ventricular function, extreme left ventricular hypertrophy, aortic stenosis). VT may degenerate suddenly into VF. Pulseless VT is treated in the same way as VF: by immediate defibrillation.

In the presence of a cardiac output, treatment of VT should follow the broad complex tachycardia algorithm described in Chapter 12.

The QRS morphology may be monomorphic or polymorphic. In monomorphic VT (Rhythm Strip 10), the rhythm is regular (or almost regular). The rate during VT may be anything from 100-300 min$^{-1}$, rarely faster. It is unusual to see more than slight variation in heart rate during any single episode of VT (other than in response to anti-arrhythmic drug therapy). Atrial activity may continue independently of ventricular activity; the identification of P waves, dissociated from QRS complexes during broad complex tachycardia, identifies the rhythm as VT. Occasionally these atrial beats

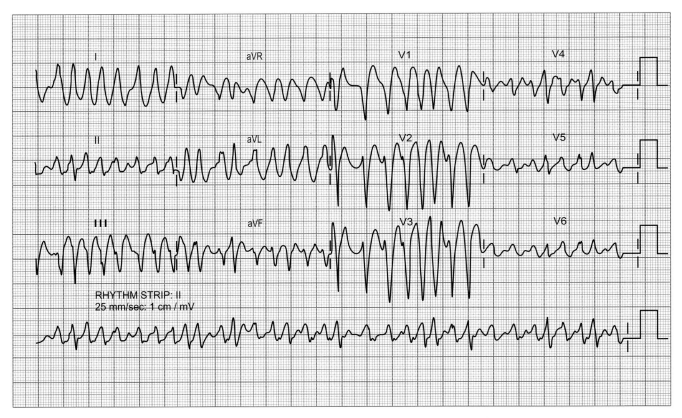

**Figure 7.9 Pre-excited atrial fibrillation in a patient with Wolff-Parkinson-White syndrome**

ALS

may be conducted to the ventricles, causing capture beats or fusion beats (Rhythm Strip 11). A capture beat produces a normal-looking QRS complex during monomorphic VT, without otherwise interrupting the arrhythmia. In a fusion beat, a wave of depolarisation travelling down from the AV node occurs simultaneously with a wave of depolarisation travelling up from the ventricular focus producing the arrhythmia. This results in a hybrid QRS complex caused by fusion of the normal QRS complex with the complex of the monomorphic VT.

In the presence of bundle branch block, a supraventricular tachycardia (SVT) will produce a broad complex tachycardia. After myocardial infarction, most broad complex tachycardia will be ventricular in origin. The safest approach is to regard all broad complex tachycardia in this setting as VT until, or unless, proved otherwise.

One important type of polymorphic VT is torsade de pointes in which the axis of the electrical activity changes in a rotational way so that the overall appearance of the ECG on a rhythm strip produces a sinusoidal pattern (Rhythm Strip 12). This arrhythmia usually arises in patients with a prolonged QT interval. This can occur as an inherited phenomenon in some families. More commonly it is caused by drugs, including some anti-arrhythmic drugs. Many patients with torsade de pointes VT are also hypokalaemic and/or hypomagnesaemic. It is important to recognise torsade de pointes VT, because effective treatment (prevention of recurrent episodes) will require removal of any predisposing causes (i.e., drugs), intravenous magnesium and correction of any other electrolyte abnormality, and may also require the use of overdrive pacing. Torsade de pointes VT can itself cause cardiac arrest (in which case it is treated by defibrillation) and can also degenerate into VF.

## Asystole

The appearance of asystole has been described already (Rhythm Strip 2). Sometimes it is not clear whether the observed rhythm is asystole or very fine VF. In this situation, immediate treatment is to provide good quality CPR and continued observation. If fine VF was present, good CPR may increase the amplitude and frequency of the VF, making that diagnosis clear and increasing the probability of successful defibrillation.

## Pulseless electrical activity

The term pulseless electrical activity (PEA) does not refer to a specific cardiac rhythm. It defines the clinical absence of cardiac output despite electrical activity that would normally be expected to produce a cardiac output. It generally has a poor prognosis especially when it is caused by a very large acute myocardial infarction. Potentially more treatable causes include massive pulmonary thromboembolism, tension pneumothorax, cardiac tamponade and acute severe blood loss.

# Peri-arrest arrhythmias

These are defined according to heart rate (bradyarrhythmia, tachyarrhythmia or arrhythmia with a normal rate), as this will dictate initial treatment (Chapter 12). In the unstable patient concentrate on early treatment to prevent deterioration, rather than on prolonged attempts to identify the precise rhythm.

## Bradyarrhythmia

A bradycardia is present when the ventricular (QRS) rate is less than 60 $min^{-1}$ (Rhythm Strip 13). Bradycardia may be a physiological state in very fit people or during sleep, or may be an expected result of treatment (e.g., with a beta-blocker). Pathological bradycardia may be caused by malfunction of the SA node or from delay in or block of atrioventricular conduction. Some patients with these rhythm abnormalities may need treatment with an implanted pacemaker (Rhythm Strip 14).

The emergency treatment of most bradycardia is with atropine and/or cardiac pacing. Occasionally it may be necessary to use sympathomimetic drugs such as adrenaline. The need for treatment depends on the haemodynamic effect of the arrhythmia and the risk of developing asystole, rather than the precise ECG classification of the bradycardia. Extreme bradycardia may sometimes precede cardiac arrest and this may be prevented by prompt and appropriate treatment. In this context the most important bradyarrhythmia is acquired complete heart block (see below).

### Heart block: first degree atrioventricular block

The PR interval is the time between the onset of the P wave and the start of the QRS complex (whether this begins with a Q wave or R wave). The normal PR interval is between 0.12 and 0.20 sec. First degree atrioventricular (AV) block is present when the PR interval is greater than 0.20 sec and is a common finding (Rhythm Strip 15). It represents a delay in conduction through the AV junction (the AV node and bundle of His). In some instances this may be physiological (for example in trained athletes). There are many other causes of first degree AV block, including primary disease (fibrosis) of the conducting system and therapy with drugs that delay conduction through the AV node. First degree AV block rarely causes any symptoms and rarely requires treatment.

### Heart block: second degree atrioventricular block

Second degree AV block is present when some, but not all, P waves are conducted to the ventricles, resulting in absence of a QRS complex after some P waves. There are two types:

ALS

### Möbitz Type I or Wenckebach AV block

The PR interval shows progressive prolongation after each successive P wave until a P wave occurs without a resulting QRS complex. Usually the cycle is then repeated (Rhythm Strip 16). Any condition that delays AV conduction can produce Wenkebach AV block. This may include ischaemia following acute myocardial infarction (especially inferior infarction). If asymptomatic, this rhythm does not usually require immediate treatment. The need for treatment is usually dictated by the risk of developing more severe AV block or asystole.

### Möbitz Type II AV block

There is a constant PR interval in the conducted beats but some of the P waves are not followed by QRS complexes. This may occur randomly, without any consistent pattern, or there may be a regular relationship between P waves and conducted QRS complexes. For example, 2:1 AV block is present if a QRS complex follows every other P wave (Rhythm Strip 17). If only every third beat is conducted the AV block is 3:1 (Rhythm Strip 18).

### Heart block: third degree atrioventricular block

In third degree (complete) AV block, there is no relationship between P waves and QRS complexes; atrial and ventricular depolarisation arises independently from separate 'pacemakers' (Rhythm Strip 19). The site of the pacemaker stimulating the ventricles will determine the ventricular rate and QRS width. A pacemaker site in the AV node or proximal bundle of His may have an intrinsic rate of 40-50 min$^{-1}$ or sometimes higher and may produce a narrow QRS complex. A pacemaker site in the distal His-Purkinje fibres or ventricular myocardium will produce broad QRS complexes, often have a rate of 30-40 min$^{-1}$ or less, and is more likely to stop abruptly, resulting in asystole.

### Escape rhythms

If the normal cardiac pacemaker (SA node) fails, or operates abnormally slowly, cardiac depolarisation may be initiated from a 'subsidiary' pacemaker in atrial myocardium, AV node, conducting fibres or ventricular myocardium. The resulting escape rhythm will usually be slower than the normal sinus rate. As indicated above, subsidiary pacemakers situated distally in the conducting system tend to produce slower heart rates than those situated more proximally. Thus a ventricular escape rhythm will usually be slower than a 'junctional' rhythm arising from the AV node or bundle of His.

The term idioventricular rhythm is used to describe a rhythm arising from ventricular myocardium. This includes ventricular escape rhythms seen in the presence of complete AV block. The term accelerated idioventricular rhythm is used to describe an idioventricular rhythm with a normal heart rate (usually faster than the sinus rate but not fast enough to be VT). This type of rhythm is observed quite frequently after successful thrombolysis for acute myocardial infarction (a 'reperfusion arrhythmia'). Accelerated idioventricular rhythms do not influence prognosis unless they cause haemodynamic compromise or develop into VT or VF, which is relatively uncommon. The QRS complex of an idioventricular rhythm will be broad (i.e., 0.12 seconds or greater), whereas a junctional rhythm may be narrow or broad, depending on whether conduction to the ventricles occurs normally, or with bundle branch block.

### Agonal rhythm

Agonal rhythm occurs in dying patients. It is characterised by the presence of slow, irregular, wide ventricular complexes, often of varying morphology (Rhythm Strip 20). This rhythm is seen commonly during the later stages of unsuccessful resuscitation attempts. The complexes slow inexorably and often become progressively broader before all recognisable activity is lost.

## Tachyarrhythmia

A pathological tachycardia may arise from atrial myocardium, the AV junction or ventricular myocardium. Sinus tachycardia is not an arrhythmia and usually represents a response to some other physiological or pathological state.

### Narrow-complex Tachycardia

When a tachycardia arises from tissue situated above the bifurcation of the bundle of His, it is described as supraventricular (Rhythm Strip 21). The QRS complexes will be narrow if ventricular depolarisation occurs normally, but will be broad if bundle branch block is present. QRS complexes may be regular in many rhythms or may be irregular in the presence of atrial fibrillation or variably conducted atrial flutter. Overall, tachycardia with narrow QRS complexes has a relatively favourable prognosis, but the outlook will vary with individual clinical circumstances. These rhythms may be tolerated poorly by patients with chronic heart disease and may provoke angina in patients with coronary heart disease.

### Atrial Fibrillation

Atrial fibrillation is the most common arrhythmia encountered in clinical practice. It characterised by disorganised electrical activity in the atria. No recognisable P waves or co-ordinated atrial activity can be seen in any lead (Rhythm Strip 6). The baseline is irregular and chaotic atrial activity is best seen in lead V1 where the atrial waveform is irregular in both amplitude and frequency. The QRS rhythm is irregularly irregular (i.e., there is no consistent R-R interval from beat to beat). The ventricular rate will depend on the refractory period of the AV junction. In the absence of treatment or pre-existing disease of the AV node, the resulting ventricular rate will be rapid, as many of the atrial impulses that arrive at the AV node will be conducted. A ventricular rate in the range of 120–180 min$^{-1}$ often results.

Causes of AF include hypertension, structural heart disease, and alcohol excess. In coronary heart disease AF usually results from left ventricular impairment (acute or chronic) and not as a direct result of ischaemia of atrial myocardium.

### Atrial Flutter

In atrial flutter, atrial activity is seen on the ECG as flutter or F waves at a rate of about 300 min[-1] (Rhythm Strip 22). These are best seen in the inferior leads II, III and aVF where they have a 'saw-tooth' appearance (Figure 7.5). The ventricular rate depends on AV conduction but there is often 2:1 (Rhythm Strip 9) or 3:1 conduction (referred to as atrial flutter with 2:1 or 3:1 block). If the block is constant the ventricular rhythm will be regular, but variable block causes an irregular ventricular rhythm. Like atrial fibrillation, atrial flutter is often, but not always, associated with underlying disease. Atrial flutter usually arises in the right atrium so is a recognised complication of diseases that affect the right heart, including chronic obstructive pulmonary disease, major pulmonary embolism, complex congenital heart disease and chronic congestive heart failure of any cause.

### Broad-complex Tachycardia

Broad-complex tachycardia may be:

- a tachycardia arising in the ventricle below the bifurcation of the bundle of His, i.e., VT (Rhythm Strip 10); or,

- a supraventricular tachycardia conducted aberrantly (right or left bundle branch block) to the ventricles.

The clinical consequences depend on:

- heart rate during the arrhythmia;

- the presence or absence of structural heart disease or coronary disease;

- duration of the arrhythmia.

Ventricular tachycardia may degenerate into VF, especially if the VT is very fast (e.g., 200 min[-1] or faster) or if the heart is unstable as a consequence of acute ischaemia or infarction, or in the presence of electrolyte abnormality (hypokalaemia or hypomagnesaemia).

Treat all broad-complex tachycardia as ventricular tachycardia unless there is good evidence that it is supraventricular in origin.

Patients with WPW syndrome have accessory pathways connecting atrial and ventricular myocardium. Some atrioventricular conduction occurs through these pathways as well as through the AV node. This results in widening of the QRS complexes by so-called delta waves. In the presence of such an accessory pathway that bypasses the AV node, AF may result in a ventricular rate that is so fast that cardiac output decreases dramatically. The ECG appearances are of a very rapid, irregular, broad complex tachycardia that usually shows variability in the width of QRS complexes. This rhythm may be mistaken for VF or misdiagnosed as irregular VT. Overall the rhythm is more organised than ventricular fibrillation and lacks the random chaotic activity of variable amplitude.

## The QT interval

When identifying and treating rhythm abnormalities it is important to recognise likely underlying causes that may influence choice of effective treatment. These may be identified from clinical assessment (e.g., myocardial infarction), laboratory tests (e.g., electrolyte abnormality) or from the ECG. Prolongation of the QT interval on the ECG may predispose to ventricular arrhythmia, in particular torsade de pointes VT and VF.

The QT interval is measured from the start of the QRS complex to the end of the T wave. It can be difficult to measure accurately, mainly because it may be difficult to identify the end of the T wave. This may be especially difficult when prominent U waves are present, merging with the end of the T wave. U waves can be a feature of some abnormalities (e.g., hypokalaemia) but may be present in some healthy people with normal hearts.

The length of the QT interval may also vary between different leads of the same ECG. This may partly reflect variation in amplitude and direction of the T wave, making it more difficult to measure in some leads than others. Variation in the QT interval (QT dispersion) has also been shown to be associated with an increased risk of death in patients with ischaemic heart disease, but this finding has not been developed into a useful measurement for use in clinical practice.

The QT interval varies with age, with gender and in particular with heart rate. The QT interval shortens as the heart rate increases. A correction can be made to allow for this, using the measured QT interval and heart rate to calculate the corrected QT interval (QTc). Many modern ECG machines measure the QT and other intervals and calculate the QTc automatically. These measurements are only accurate if the ECG recording is of good quality. Most ECG machines cannot distinguish between T waves and U waves. Always look at the recording and make sure that the quoted measurements are not obviously inaccurate.

Abnormality of the QT interval can be seen in various situations. Hypercalcaemia and digoxin shorten it. Hypokalaemia, hypomagnesaemia, hypocalcaemia, hypothermia and myocarditis can all cause QT prolongation. There is also a long list of drugs that may prolong the QT interval, including class I and class III anti-arrhythmic drugs.

There are several genetic abnormalities in which the QT interval is prolonged or there is abnormality of ventricular repolarisation (principally the long QT and Brugada

ALS

syndromes). The abnormality of repolarisation places them at risk of ventricular arrhythmia and sudden death. Some of these patients require an implantable cardioverter-defibrillator to protect against this. It is especially important that patients with these syndromes are not given any drug that may cause further QT prolongation.

## Key learning points

- A systematic approach to ECG rhythm analysis enables accurate assessment of any rhythm abnormality sufficiently to enable safe, effective treatment.

- Recordings of any rhythm abnormality and of the ECG in sinus rhythm provide valuable diagnostic information and help the correct choice of longer-term treatment.

- Accurate monitoring of the cardiac rhythm is essential for any patient at high risk of developing life-threatening arrhythmia.

- Accurate monitoring of the cardiac rhythm is essential in the management of cardiac arrest.

## Further reading

Blomstrom-Lundqvist C, Scheinmann M M et al. American College of Cardiology/American Heart Association Task Force and the European Society of Cardiology Committee for Practice Guidelines. ACC/AHA/ESC Guidelines for the Management of Patients With Supraventricular Arrhythmias. European Heart Journal 2003;24:1857-1897.

Fuster V, Lyden R E et al. American College of Cardiology/American Heart Association Task Force and the European Society of Cardiology Committee for Practice Guidelines and Policy Conferences. ACC/AHA/ESC guidelines for the management of patients with atrial fibrillation. European Heart Journal 2001; 22:1852-1923.

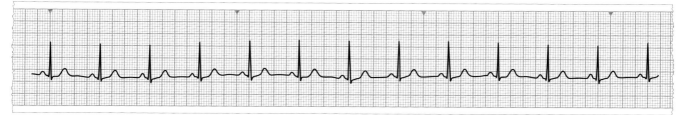

**Rhythm Strip 1. Normal sinus rhythm**

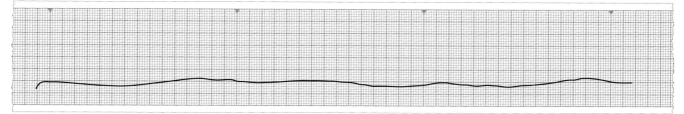

**Rhythm Strip 2. Asystole**

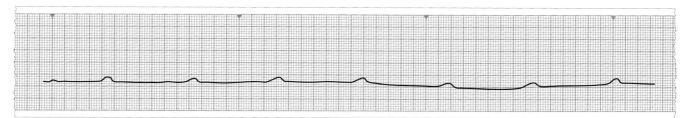

**Rhythm Strip 3. P-wave asystole**

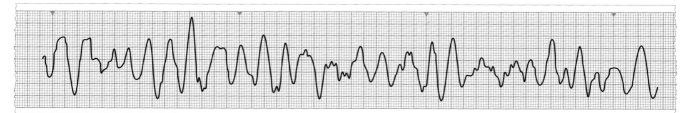

**Rhythm Strip 4. Course ventricular fibrillation**

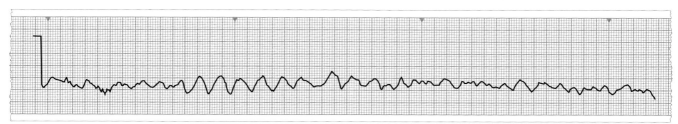

**Rhythm Strip 5. Fine ventricular fibrillation**

ALS

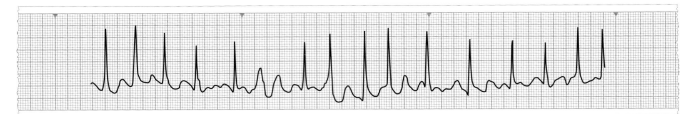

**Rhythm Strip 6. Atrial fibrillation**

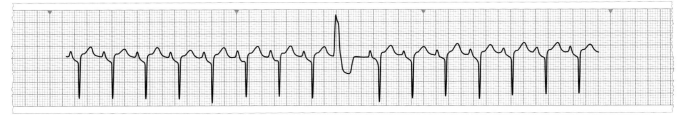

**Rhythm Strip 7. Premature ventricular beat**

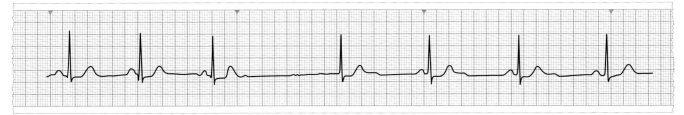

**Rhythm Strip 8. Junctional escape beat**

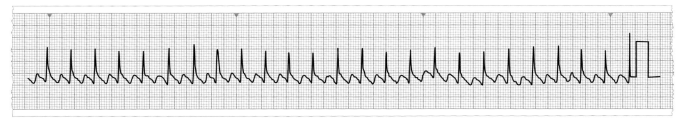

**Rhythm Strip 9. Atrial flutter with 2:1 atrioventricular block**

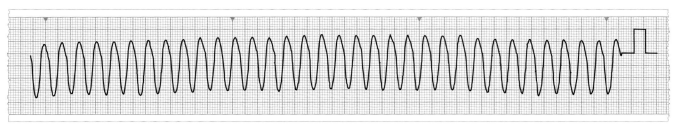

**Rhythm Strip 10. Monomorphic ventricular tachycardia**

ALS

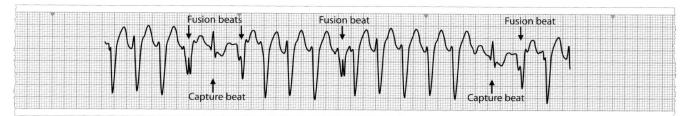

**Rhythm Strip 11. Ventricular tachycardia with capture and fusion beats**

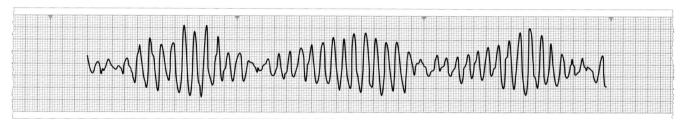

**Rhythm Strip 12. Torsade de pointes**

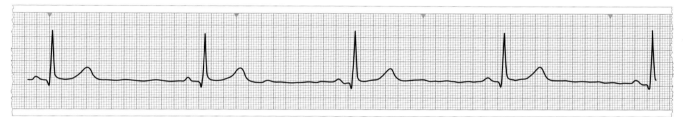

**Rhythm Strip 13. Sinus bradycardia**

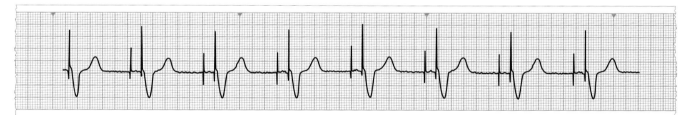

**Rhythm Strip 14. Paced rhythm**

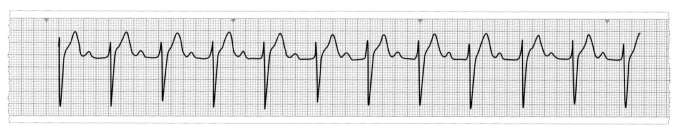

**Rhythm Strip 15. First degree atrioventricular block**

ALS

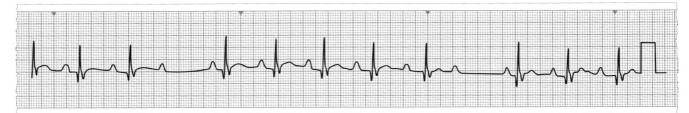

**Rhythm Strip 16. Mobitz type I or Wenckebach block**

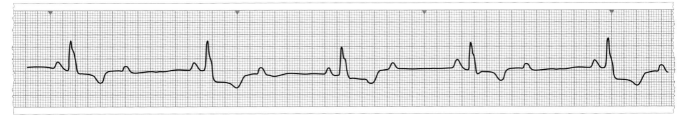

**Rhythm Strip 17. Mobitz type II second degree atrioventricular block (2:1)**

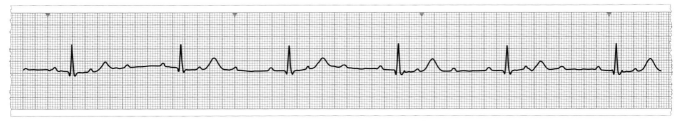

**Rhythm Strip 18. Mobitz type II second degree atrioventricular block (3:1)**

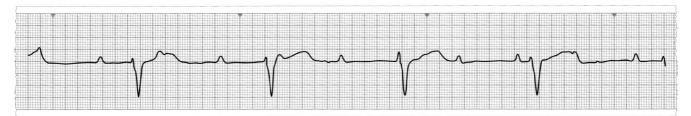

**Rhythm Strip 19. Third degree (complete) atrioventricular block**

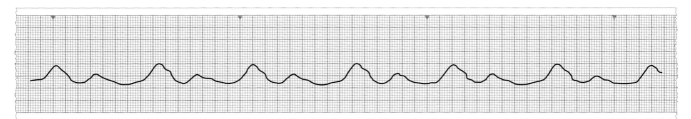

**Rhythm Strip 20. Agonal rhythm**

ALS

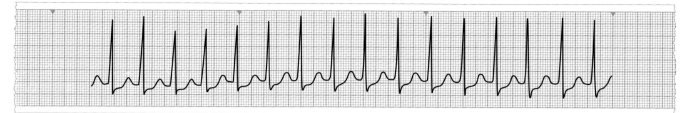

**Rhythm Strip 21. Supraventricular tachycardia**

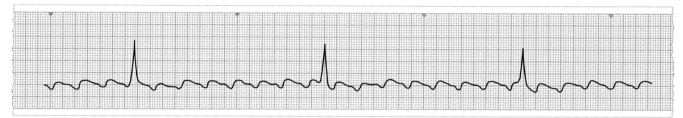

**Rhythm Strip 22. Atrial flutter with a high degree of atrioventricular block**

**ALS**

# Defibrillation

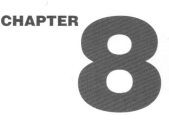

## Introduction

Following the onset of ventricular fibrillation / pulseless ventricular tachycardia (VF/VT), cardiac output ceases and cerebral hypoxic injury starts within 3 min. If complete neurological recovery is to be achieved, early successful defibrillation with a return of spontaneous circulation (ROSC) is needed. Defibrillation is a key link in the chain of survival and is one of the few interventions that has been shown to improve outcome from VF/VT cardiac arrest. The probability of successful defibrillation and subsequent survival to hospital discharge declines rapidly with time and the ability to deliver early defibrillation is one of the most important factors in determining survival from cardiac arrest. For every minute that passes between collapse and attempted defibrillation, mortality increases 7-10% in the absence of bystander CPR. The shorter the interval between the onset of VF/VT and delivery of the shock, the greater the chance of successful defibrillation and survival. If there is any delay in obtaining a defibrillator, start chest compressions and ventilation immediately. When bystander CPR is provided, the decrease in survival is more gradual and averages 3-4% per minute from collapse to defibrillation. CPR can double or triple survival from witnessed cardiac arrest at any interval to defibrillation.

## Mechanism of defibrillation

Defibrillation is the passage of current of sufficient magnitude across the myocardium to depolarise a critical mass of the cardiac muscle simultaneously, to enable the natural pacemaker tissue to resume control. Success is defined as termination of fibrillation or, more precisely, the absence of VF/VT at 5 sec after shock delivery, although the ultimate goal is ROSC. To achieve this, all defibrillators have three features in common: a power source capable of providing direct current, a capacitor that can be charged to a pre-determined energy level and two electrodes which are placed on the patient's chest through which the capacitor is discharged.

Success depends on sufficient current being delivered to the myocardium. However, the delivered current is difficult to determine because it is influenced by transthoracic

impedance and electrode position. Furthermore, much of the current is diverted along other pathways in the thorax away from the heart and as little as 4% reaches the heart. Some defibrillators can measure the transthoracic impedance and adjust their output accordingly (impedance compensation).

There is no definite relationship between body size and energy requirements for defibrillation in adults. Although other factors such as the patient's metabolic state, extent of myocardial ischaemia, and previous drug therapy influence the success of defibrillation attempts, they cannot usually be modified during cardiopulmonary resuscitation.

## Factors affecting defibrillation success

### Transthoracic impedance

Defibrillation technique must be optimised to minimise the transthoracic impedance and maximise delivery of current to the myocardium. In adults, impedance is normally in the range 70-80 ohm, but in the presence of poor technique may rise to 150 ohm, halving the current delivered and thereby reducing the chance of successful defibrillation. Transthoracic impedance is influenced by electrode-to-skin contact, electrode or paddle size, the paddle-skin coupling material, paddle force, and phase of ventilation. The presence of a transdermal drug patch on the patient's chest may prevent good contact and may cause arcing and burns if paddles or electrodes are placed over them; remove them and wipe the area dry before applying the electrodes and attempting defibrillation.

### Shaving the chest

It is often difficult to obtain good electrode-to-skin contact in patients with hairy chests. This increases impedance, reduces defibrillation efficacy and may cause burns to the patient's chest. If a razor is available immediately use it to remove hair from the area where the electrodes are placed. However, defibrillation should not be delayed if a razor is not to hand immediately.

### Electrode size

The sum of the electrode areas should be a minimum of 150 cm$^2$. Larger electrodes have lower impedance, but excessively large electrodes may result in less transmyocardial current flow. For adult defibrillation, both handheld paddle electrodes and self-adhesive pad electrodes 8-12 cm in diameter are used and function well.

### Coupling agents

If using manual paddles, gel pads are preferable to electrode pastes and gels because the latter can spread between the two paddles, creating the potential for a spark. Do not use bare electrodes without a coupling material because this causes high transthoracic impedance and may increase the severity of any cutaneous burns. Do not use medical gels or pastes of poor electrical conductivity (e.g., ultrasound gel).

## Paddle force

If using paddles, apply them firmly to the chest wall. This reduces transthoracic impedance by improving electrical contact at the electrode-skin interface and reducing thoracic volume. The defibrillator operator should always press firmly on handheld electrode paddles, the optimal force being 8 kg in an adult. An 8-kg force may be attainable only by the strongest members of the cardiac arrest team.

# Electrode position

No human studies have evaluated the electrode position as a determinant of ROSC or survival from VF/VT cardiac arrest. Transmyocardial current during defibrillation is likely to be maximal when the electrodes are placed so that the area of the heart that is fibrillating lies directly between them (i.e., ventricles in VF/VT, atria in AF). Therefore, the optimal electrode position may not be the same for ventricular and atrial arrhythmias.

When attempting to defibrillate a patient in VF/VT, the standard procedure is to place one electrode to the right of the upper sternum below the clavicle. The apical paddle is placed in the mid-axillary line, approximately level with the V6 ECG electrode or female breast. This position should be clear of any breast tissue. It is important that this electrode is placed sufficiently laterally (Figure 8.1). Although the electrodes are marked positive and negative, each can be placed in either position. Other acceptable pad positions include:

- Placement of each electrode on the lateral chest walls, one on the right and the other on the left side (bi-axillary).

- One electrode anteriorly, over the left precordium, and the other electrode on the back behind the heart, just inferior to the left scapula.

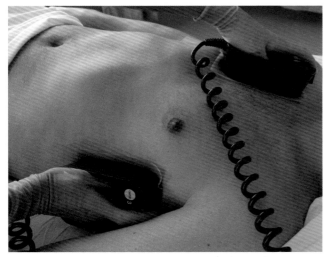

**Figure 8.1 Standard electrode positions for defibrillation**

- Asymmetrically shaped apical electrodes have lower impedance when placed longitudinally rather than transversely. Orientate the long axis of the apical paddle in a cranio-caudal direction.

## Pads versus paddles

Self-adhesive defibrillation pads are safe and effective and are preferable to standard defibrillation paddles. Consider using self-adhesive pads in peri-arrest situations and in clinical situations where patient access is difficult. They have similar transthoracic impedance (and therefore efficacy) to manual paddles and enable the operator to defibrillate the patient from a safe distance rather than leaning over the patient. When used for initial monitoring of a rhythm, both pads and paddles enable quicker delivery of the first shock compared with standard ECG electrodes, but self-adhesive pads are quicker than paddles.

When gel pads are used with paddles, the electrolyte gel becomes polarised and can be a poor conductor after defibrillation. This can cause spurious asystole that may persist for 3-4 min when used to monitor the rhythm; a phenomenon not reported with self-adhesive pads. When using a gel pad/paddle combination, confirm a diagnosis of asystole with independent ECG electrodes rather than the paddles.

# One shock versus three-shock sequence

There are no published human or animal studies comparing a single-shock protocol with a three-stacked shock protocol for treatment of VF cardiac arrest. Animal studies show that relatively short interruptions in external chest compression to deliver rescue breaths or perform rhythm analysis are associated with post-resuscitation myocardial dysfunction and reduced survival. Interruptions in external chest compression also reduce the chances of converting VF to another rhythm. Analysis of CPR performance during out-of-hospital and in-hospital cardiac arrest has shown that significant interruptions are common.

With first-shock efficacy of biphasic waveforms exceeding 90%, failure to cardiovert VF successfully suggests the need for a period of CPR rather than a further shock. Thus, immediately after giving a single shock, and without reassessing the rhythm or feeling for a pulse, resume CPR (30 compressions:2 ventilations) for 2 min before delivering another shock (if indicated) (see below). Even if the defibrillation attempt is successful in restoring a perfusing rhythm, it is very rare for a pulse to be palpable immediately after defibrillation and the delay in trying to palpate a pulse will further compromise the myocardium if a perfusing rhythm has not been restored. If a perfusing rhythm has been restored, giving chest compressions does not increase the chance of VF recurring. In the presence of post-shock asystole chest compressions may induce VF.

This single shock strategy is applicable to both monophasic and biphasic defibrillators.

# Shock energy and waveforms

Although energy levels are selected for defibrillation, it is the transmyocardial current flow that achieves defibrillation. Current correlates well with successful defibrillation and cardioversion. The optimal current for defibrillation using a monophasic waveform is in the range of 30-40 A. Indirect evidence from measurements during cardioversion for atrial fibrillation suggests that the current during defibrillation using biphasic waveforms is in the range of 15-20 A.

The optimal energy dose for defibrillation is that which achieves defibrillation and ROSC whilst causing the minimum myocardial injury. Use of an appropriate energy dose also reduces the number of repetitive shocks, which in turn limits myocardial injury.

## Monophasic defibrillators

Monophasic defibrillators are no longer manufactured although many remain in use. These devices deliver a current that flows in one direction. There are two main monophasic waveform shapes: a damped sinusoidal waveform falls to zero gradually (Figure 8.2), and a truncated exponential waveform falls instantaneously. In the past, the first and second monophasic shocks used for defibrillation were at a lower energy (200 J) than subsequent shocks (360 J). Because of the lower efficacy of the monophasic waveform compared with the biphasic waveform, the recommended initial energy level for the first shock using a monophasic defibrillator is now 360 J. Although higher energy doses risk causing more myocardial injury, the benefits of earlier conversion to a perfusing rhythm are paramount. The use of single shocks instead of three-stacked shocks also makes it important to maximise the efficacy of the first shock. If the first shock is unsuccessful, give the second and subsequent shocks at 360 J.

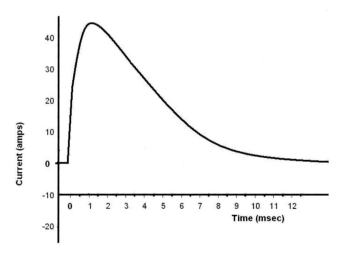

**Figure 8.2 A monophasic damped sinusoidal waveform**

## Biphasic defibrillators

Biphasic waveforms deliver current that flows in a positive direction for a specified duration before reversing to a negative direction for the remainder of the electrical discharge. There are two main types of biphasic waveform: the biphasic truncated exponential (BTE) (Figure 8.3) and rectilinear biphasic (RLB) (Figure 8.4). Some biphasic defibrillators compensate for the wide variations in transthoracic impedance by electronically adjusting the waveform magnitude and duration. The optimal ratio of first-phase to second-phase duration has not been established and whether different waveforms have differing efficacy for VF of differing durations is also unknown.

First-shock efficacy for long duration VF/VT is greater with biphasic (86-98%) than monophasic waveforms (54-91%) and therefore use of the former is recommended whenever possible. Biphasic defibrillation requires less energy and hence these devices have smaller capacitors, need less battery power, and waveform shape can be controlled by solid-state circuitry without the need for an inductor. Consequently they are smaller, lighter and easily portable.

There is no evidence that one biphasic waveform or device is more effective than another. Although the initial biphasic shock energy should be no lower than 120 J for a RLB waveform and 150 J for BTE waveforms, it is recommended that the initial biphasic shock should be at least 150 J whatever the waveform.

If the provider is unaware of the effective dose range of the device, use a dose of 200 J for the first shock. This 200 J default energy has been chosen because it falls within the reported range of selected doses that are effective for first and subsequent biphasic shocks and can be provided by every biphasic manual defibrillator available today.

If the first shock is unsuccessful, second and subsequent shocks can be delivered using either fixed or escalating energies (150-360 J), depending on the device in use. If the provider is unaware of the effective dose range of the biphasic device and a default 200 J dose has been given for the first shock, use either an equal or higher dose for second or subsequent shocks, depending on the capabilities of the device.

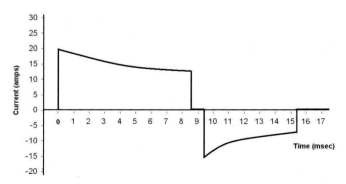

**Figure 8.3 Biphasic truncated exponential waveform**

ALS

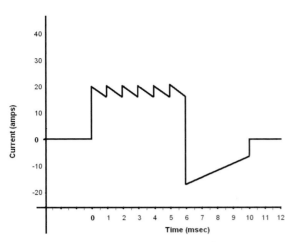

**Figure 8.4 Rectilinear biphasic waveform**

### Recurrent ventricular fibrillation

If a shockable rhythm recurs after successful defibrillation (with or without ROSC), give the next shock with the energy level that had previously been successful.

## Safety

Attempted defibrillation should be undertaken without risk to members of the resuscitation team. Be wary of wet surroundings or clothing – wipe any water from the patient's chest before attempted defibrillation. No part of any person should make direct or indirect contact with the patient. Do not hold intravenous infusion equipment or the patient's trolley during shock delivery. The defibrillator operator must not touch any part of the electrode surface, and electrode gel must not spread across the surface of the chest. Gel-impregnated pads reduce this risk – use them whenever possible. The operator must ensure that everyone is clear of the patient before delivering a shock.

## Safe use of oxygen during defibrillation

In an oxygen-enriched atmosphere, sparking from poorly applied defibrillator paddles can cause a fire. There are several reports of fires being caused in this way and most have resulted in significant burns to the patient. The risk of fire during attempted defibrillation can be minimised by taking the following precautions:

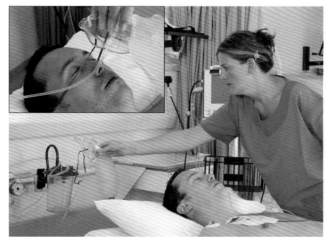

**Figure 8.5 Removal of oxygen mask before defibrillation**

- Take off any oxygen mask or nasal cannulae and place them at least 1 m away from the patient's chest (Figure 8.5).

- Leave the ventilation bag connected to the tracheal tube or other airway adjunct. When a ventilation bag is left attached to a tracheal tube, no increase in oxygen concentration occurs in the zone of defibrillation, even with an oxygen flow of 15 l min⁻¹. Alternatively, disconnect the ventilation bag from the tracheal tube (or other airway adjunct such as the laryngeal mask airway, Combitube or Laryngeal Tube), and remove it at least 1 m from the patient's chest during defibrillation.

- If the patient is connected to a ventilator, for example in the operating room or critical care unit, leave the ventilator tubing (breathing circuit) connected to the tracheal tube unless chest compressions prevent the ventilator from delivering adequate tidal volumes. In this case, the ventilator is usually substituted by a ventilation bag, which can be left connected or detached and removed to a distance of at least 1 m. If the ventilator tubing is disconnected, ensure that it is kept at least 1 m from the patient or, better still, switch the ventilator off; modern ventilators generate massive oxygen flows when disconnected. During normal use, when connected to a tracheal tube, oxygen from a ventilator in the critical care unit will be vented from the main ventilator housing well away from the defibrillation zone. Patients in the critical care unit may be dependent on positive end expiratory pressure (PEEP) to maintain adequate oxygenation; during cardioversion, when the spontaneous circulation potentially enables blood to remain well oxygenated, it is particularly appropriate to leave the critically ill patient connected to the ventilator during shock delivery.

- Minimise the risk of sparks during defibrillation. Theoretically, self-adhesive defibrillation pads are less likely to cause sparks than manual paddles.

### Safety when using defibrillator paddles

Charge a manual defibrillator only with the paddles on the patient's chest, not whilst they are held in the air. When the paddles are first placed on the patient's chest, inform team members whether the paddles are about to be charged or are being used simply to monitor the heart rhythm. If the defibrillator is charged, but a shock is no longer indicated, modern equipment enables the charge to be discharged safely by altering the energy setting.

## Automated external defibrillators

Automated external defibrillators are sophisticated, reliable computerised devices that use voice and visual prompts to guide lay rescuers and healthcare professionals to attempt defibrillation safely in cardiac arrest victims (Figure 8.6). Advances in technology, particularly with respect to battery capacity, and software arrhythmia analysis have enabled the mass production of relatively cheap, reliable and easily operated portable defibrillators. Shock-advisory defibrillators have ECG-analysis capability but can be manually over-riden by healthcare providers capable of rhythm recognition.

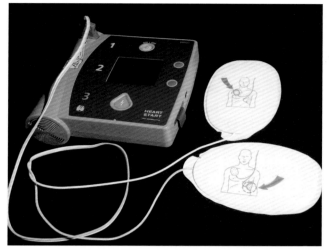

**Figure 8.6 An automated external defibrillator**

## Automated rhythm analysis

Automated external defibrillators have microprocessors that analyse several features of the ECG, including frequency and amplitude. Some AEDs are programmed to detect spontaneous movement by the patient or others. Developing technology should soon enable AEDs to provide information about frequency and depth of chest compressions during CPR that may improve resuscitation performance by all rescuers.

Automated external defibrillators have been tested extensively against libraries of recorded cardiac rhythms and in many trials in adults and children. They are extremely accurate in rhythm analysis. Although AEDs are not designed to deliver synchronised shocks, all AEDs will recommend shocks for VT if the rate and R-wave morphology exceed preset values.

## In-hospital use of AEDs

Two non-randomised studies of adults with in-hospital cardiac arrest from shockable rhythms showed higher survival-to–hospital discharge rates when defibrillation was provided through an AED program than with manual defibrillation alone.

Delayed defibrillation may occur when patients sustain cardiac arrest in unmonitored hospital beds and in outpatient departments. In these areas several minutes may elapse before resuscitation teams arrive with a defibrillator and deliver shocks. Despite limited evidence, AEDs should be considered for the hospital setting as a way to facilitate defibrillation as soon as possible (within 3 min of collapse at the most) especially in areas where staff have no rhythm recognition skills or where they use defibrillators infrequently. An effective system for training and retraining should be in place. Adequate numbers of staff should be trained to enable achievement of the goal of providing the first shock within 3 min of collapse anywhere in the hospital.

Training in the use of these machines can be achieved much more rapidly and easily than for manual defibrillators. Automated equipment has made attempted defibrillation

available to a much wider range of medical, nursing, paramedical, and lay workers (e.g., police and first-aiders – 'first-responder defibrillation'). Healthcare providers with a duty to perform CPR should be trained, equipped, and authorised to perform defibrillation. First-responder attempted defibrillation is vital, as the delay to delivery of the first shock is the main determinant of survival in cardiac arrest.

## Importance of uninterrupted chest compressions

The importance of early, uninterrupted external chest compression is emphasised throughout this manual. The rescuer providing chest compressions should interrupt chest compressions only for rhythm analysis and shock delivery, and should be prepared to resume chest compressions as soon as a shock is delivered. When two rescuers are present, the rescuer operating the AED should apply the electrodes whilst CPR is in progress. Interrupt CPR only when it is necessary to assess the rhythm and deliver a shock. The AED operator should be prepared to deliver a shock as soon as analysis is complete and the shock is advised, ensuring that all rescuers are not in contact with the victim. The single rescuer should practice co-ordination of CPR with efficient AED operation.

## Public access defibrillation (PAD) programmes

Public access defibrillation (PAD) and first responder AED programmes may increase the number of victims who receive bystander CPR and early defibrillation, thus improving survival from out-of-hospital cardiac arrest. These programmes require an organised and practised response with rescuers trained and equipped to recognise emergencies, activate the EMS system, provide CPR, and use the AED. Lay rescuer AED programmes with very rapid response times in airports, on aircraft, or in casinos, and uncontrolled studies using police officers as first responders have achieved reported survival rates as high as 49-74%.

Recommended elements for PAD programmes include:

- a planned and practised response;

- training of anticipated rescuers in CPR and use of the AED;

- link with the local EMS system;

- programme of continuous audit (quality improvement).

Public access defibrillation programmes are most likely to improve survival from cardiac arrest if they are established in locations where witnessed cardiac arrest is likely to occur. Suitable sites might include those where the probability of cardiac arrest occurring is at least once in every two years (e.g., airports, casinos, sports facilities). Approximately 80% of out-of-hospital cardiac arrests occur in private or residential settings; this fact inevitably limits the overall impact that PAD programmes can have on survival rates.

# Algorithm for use of an automated external defibrillator (AED)

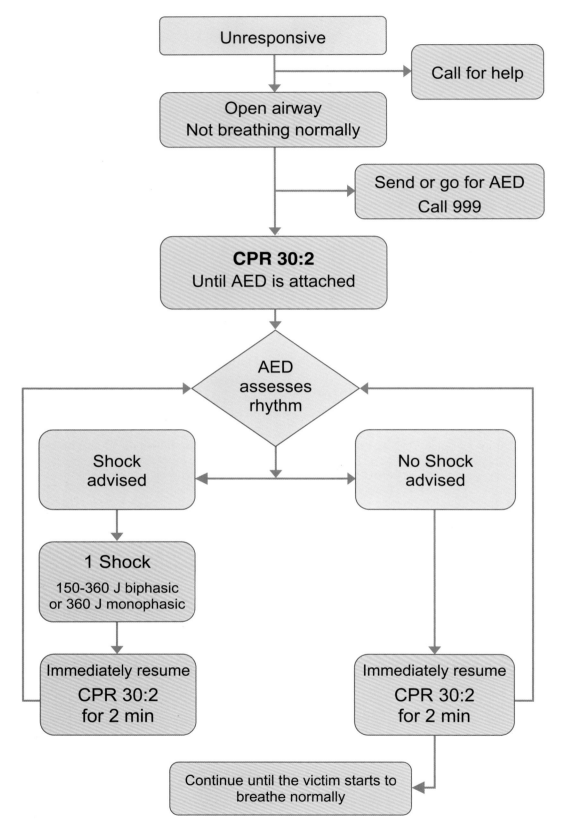

**Figure 8.7 Algorithm for the management of cardiac arrest using an AED**

ALS

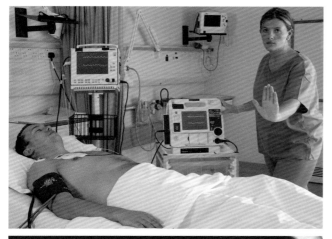

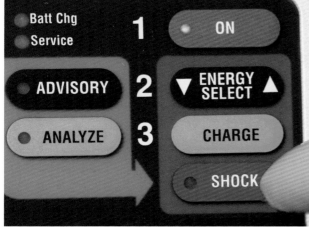

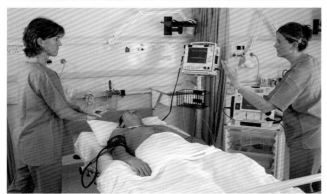

**Figure 8.8 a-c Operation of a defibrillator and efficient CPR**

## Sequence for use of an AED or shock-advisory defibrillator (Figure 8.7)

1   Make sure the victim, any bystanders, and you are safe

2   If the victim is unresponsive and not breathing normally:

   - Send someone for the AED and call for an ambulance or resuscitation team. If you are on your own, do this yourself.

3   Start CPR according to the guidelines (Chapter 4).

4   As soon as the AED arrives:

   - Switch on the AED and attach the electrode pads. If more than one rescuer is present, continue CPR while this is done.

   - Follow the voice/visual directions.

   - Ensure that nobody touches the victim whilst the AED is analysing the rhythm.

5A If a shock **IS** indicated:

   - Ensure that nobody touches the victim (Figure 8.8a).

   - Push the shock button (Figure 8.8b) as directed – fully-automatic AEDs will deliver the shock automatically.

   - Continue as directed by the voice/visual prompts.

5B If **NO** shock is indicated:

   - Immediately resume CPR using a ratio of 30 compressions to 2 rescue breaths (Figure 8.8c).

   - Continue as directed by the voice/visual prompts.

6   Continue to follow the AED prompts until:

   - Qualified help (e.g., ambulance or resuscitation team) arrives and takes over.

   - The victim starts to breathe normally, or

   - You become exhausted.

### Notes

- The carrying case with the AED must contain some strong scissors for cutting through clothing and a disposable razor for shaving chest hair in order to obtain good electrode contact.

- If ALS providers are using the AED, they should implement other ALS interventions (intubation, ventilation, IV access, drug delivery, etc.) according to local protocols.

## Manual defibrillation

Manual defibrillators (Figure 8.9) have several advantages over AEDs. They enable the operator to diagnose the rhythm and deliver a shock rapidly without having to wait for rhythm analysis. This minimises the interruption in chest compressions. Manual defibrillators often have additional facilities, such as the ability to deliver synchronised shocks, and external pacing facilities. The main disadvantage of these devices is that the operator has to be skilled in ECG rhythm recognition; therefore, in comparison with AEDs, extra training is required.

### Sequence for use of a manual defibrillator

This sequence is an integral part of the advanced life support treatment algorithm in Chapter 5.

1.   Confirm cardiac arrest – check breathing and pulse simultaneously.

2.   Confirm VF from ECG monitor or from adhesive pads or the defibrillator paddles.

ALS

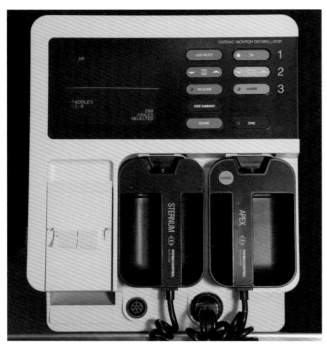

**Figure 8.9 A manual defibrillator**

3. Place self-adhesive pads or defibrillator gel pads on the patient's chest - one below the right clavicle, one in the V6 position in the midaxillary line. If more than one rescuer is present, CPR should be continued whilst this is done.

4. If using defibrillator paddles, place them firmly on gel pads (Figure 8.10).

5. Select the correct energy level: 150-200 J biphasic (360 J monophasic) for the first shock and 150-360 J biphasic (360 J monophasic) for subsequent shocks.

6. Ensure that high flow oxygen is not passing across the zone of defibrillation.

7. Warn everyone to "stand clear", and charge self-adhesive pads or defibrillator paddles.

8. Perform a quick visual check to ensure that everyone is clear.

9. Deliver the shock.

10. Minimise the interval between stopping compressions and delivering a shock; it should certainly not exceed 10 sec.

11. If using defibrillator paddles, replace them in the defibrillator.

12. Without reassessing the rhythm or feeling for a pulse, start CPR using a ratio of 30:2, starting with chest compressions.

13. Continue CPR for 2 min, then pause briefly to check the monitor.

14. If VF/VT, repeat steps 4-12 above and deliver a second shock.

15. Continue CPR for two min, then pause briefly to check the monitor.

16. If VF/VT persists give adrenaline 1 mg IV followed by third shock and 2 min CPR.

17. Repeat this sequence if VF/VT persists.

18. Give further adrenaline 1 mg IV after alternate shocks (i.e., approximately every 3-5 min).

19. After 3 shocks consider amiodarone 300 mg IV.

20. If organised electrical activity is seen during the pause to check the monitor, feel for a pulse:

    a. If a pulse is present, start post-resuscitation care.

    b. If no pulse is present, continue CPR and switch to the non-shockable algorithm.

21. If asystole is seen, continue CPR and switch to the non-shockable algorithm.

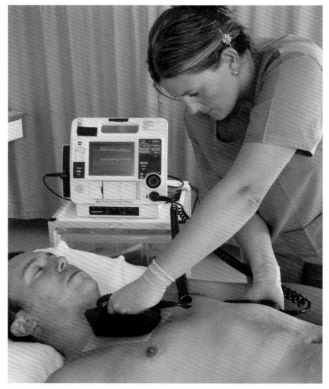

**Figure 8.10 Place defibrillator paddles firmly on gel pads**

## Prehospital defibrillation

Although previous guidelines have recommended immediate defibrillation for all shockable rhythms, recent studies of prehospital cardiac arrest suggest that a period of CPR before defibrillation may be beneficial after prolonged collapse.

Emergency medical services (EMS) personnel should give a period of about 2 min of CPR before defibrillation in patients with prolonged collapse (> 5 min). The duration of collapse is frequently difficult to estimate accurately and it may be simplest if EMS personnel are instructed to provide this period of CPR before attempted defibrillation in any cardiac arrest that they have not witnessed.

Laypeople and first responders using AEDS should attach the device as soon as possible and follow the prompts.

There is no evidence to support or refute CPR before defibrillation for in-hospital cardiac arrest. Deliver a shock as soon as possible following in-hospital cardiac arrest.

## Synchronised cardioversion

If electrical cardioversion is used to convert atrial or ventricular tachyarrhythmias, the shock must be synchronised to occur with the R wave of the electrocardiogram rather than with the T wave. By avoiding the relative refractory period, the risk of inducing VF is minimised. Most manual defibrillators incorporate a switch that enables the shock to be triggered by the R wave on the electrocardiogram. Electrodes are applied to the chest wall and cardioversion is carried out in the same way as attempted defibrillation but the operator must anticipate the slight delay between pressing the buttons and the discharge of the shock when the next R wave occurs. The defibrillator electrodes must not be moved during this lag period otherwise the QRS complex will not be detected.

Synchronisation can be difficult in VT because of the wide-complex and variable forms of ventricular arrhythmia. If synchronisation fails, give unsynchronised shocks to the unstable patient in VT to avoid prolonged delay in restoring sinus rhythm. Ventricular fibrillation or pulseless VT requires unsynchronised shocks. Conscious patients must be anaesthetised or sedated before attempting synchronised cardioversion.

With some defibrillators, the synchronised mode has to be reset if a second shock is required. Other machines remain in the synchronised mode; be careful not to leave the synchronisation switch in the 'on' position following use as this will inhibit discharge of the defibrillator when it is next used for treating VF/VT.

Energy doses for cardioversion are discussed in Chapter 12.

## Cardiac pacemakers and implantable cardioverter-defibrillators

If the patient has a cardiac pacemaker or implantable cardioverter-defibrillator (ICD), be careful when placing the electrodes. Although modern pacemakers are fitted with protection circuits, the current may travel along the pacemaker wire or ICD lead causing burns where the electrode tip makes contact with the myocardium. This may increase resistance at the contact point and gradually increase the threshold for pacing over a considerable length of time. Place the defibrillator electrodes at least 12-15 cm from the pacemaker unit to minimise the risk. If resuscitation is successful following defibrillation, check the pacemaker threshold regularly over the next two months.

## Key learning points

- For the patient in ventricular fibrillation early defibrillation is the only effective means of restoring a spontaneous circulation.

- When using a defibrillator, keep interruptions of chest compressions to an absolute minimum.

- Modern, biphasic defibrillators have a high first-shock efficacy; use single shocks interspersed with 2 min of CPR at 30:2.

## Further reading

International Liaison Committee on Resuscitation. Part 3. Defibrillation. 2005 International Consensus on Cardiopulmonary Resuscitation and Emergency Cardiovascular Care Science with Treatment Recommendations. Resuscitation 2005;67:203-211.

International Liaison Committee on Resuscitation. Part 4. Advanced Life Support. 2005 International Consensus on Cardiopulmonary Resuscitation and Emergency Cardiovascular Care Science with Treatment Recommendations. Resuscitation 2005;67:213-247.

Deakin CD, Nolan JP. European Resuscitation Council Guidelines for Resuscitation 2005. Section 3: Electrical therapies: automated external defibrillators, defibrillation, cardioversion and pacing. Resuscitation 2005;67 Suppl 1:S25-37.

Nolan JP, Deakin CD, Soar J, Bottiger BW, Smith G. European Resuscitation Council Guidelines for Resuscitation 2005. Section 4: Adult advanced life support. Resuscitation 2005;67 Suppl 1:S39-86.

ALS

ALS

# Drug Delivery

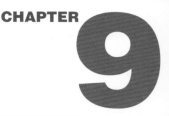

## CHAPTER 9

## Objectives

To understand:

▶ **Reasons for requiring venous access during resuscitation.**

▶ **Equipment available to obtain venous access.**

▶ **Techniques for cannulation of the central veins.**

▶ **Advantages and disadvantages of peripheral and central venous cannulation.**

▶ **Potential complications arising from intravenous cannulation.**

▶ **Use of the intraosseous and tracheal route for drug delivery.**

## Introduction

During cardiopulmonary resuscitation, access to the circulation is required for the following procedures:

- giving drugs;
- giving fluids;
- taking blood samples;
- transvenous pacing.

The intravenous route is most widely used during advanced life support, but when this fails the tracheal or intraosseous routes can be used to give drugs.

## Intravenous access

The intravenous route is the most reliable for giving drugs during resuscitation. If an intravenous cannula is already in place and its patency has been confirmed, use it first. When cannulation of a vein is necessary, the choice of using a peripheral or central vein is determined by the skill and experience of the operator and the availability of equipment. When CPR is in progress, the circulation time from the central veins (subclavian or internal jugular), through the heart to the femoral artery is approximately 30 sec compared with up to 5 min when a peripheral vein is used. Thus, if a central venous cannula is already in situ it is the preferred route for drug delivery. In the absence of a cannulated central vein, insertion of a peripheral venous cannula will be most convenient and faster; however, if a peripheral vein is used for giving a drug, follow it with a flush of intravenous fluid and raise the limb to speed up delivery to the central circulation.

## Equipment

A variety of devices can be used to obtain venous access. Two scales indicate the bore of these intravascular devices:

- Standard Wire Gauge -often referred to as the gauge (G) – the diameter of the cannula increases as the gauge size decreases;

- French Gauge (FG) - the diameter of the cannula increases as the gauge size increases.

The length of the cannula usually increases with increasing diameter.

### Cannula-over-needle

This is a popular device for achieving intravenous access. It is available in several sizes and can be used for both peripheral and central venous access. All cannulae have a standard Luer-lock fitting for attaching a giving set and some have a valved injection port through which drugs can be injected.

### Seldinger type

This equipment is used predominantly for catheterisation of the central veins. A relatively small needle is used to puncture a vein and introduce a blunt, flexible guidewire. After dilation, a larger catheter is then inserted over the guidewire into the vein. This method enables the insertion of a large-diameter catheter (e.g., 12-14 G, 7-8.5 FG) without having to use a large-diameter needle and risk damaging the vein or other adjacent structures. A similar but smaller device is available for peripheral venous cannulation.

## Access via the peripheral veins

The superficial peripheral veins in the upper limbs are used most commonly (Figure 9.1). The external jugular vein in the neck is an excellent alternative and is often prominent in patients during a cardiac arrest. The femoral vein also enables faster delivery of drugs to the heart than more peripheral veins.

The size of cannula used will depend upon its purpose. Large-diameter cannulae are required for rapid fluid administration. Secure the cannula well - it can be displaced easily during resuscitation. Use universal precautions (especially gloves); place used needles into a sharps container immediately.

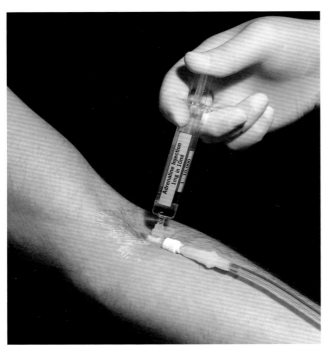

**Figure 9.1 Injection through a peripheral intravenous cannula**

### External jugular vein

In the neck, the external jugular vein is easily identified and accessible. It runs down and forward from the angle of the mandible and passes behind the middle of the clavicle (Figure 9.2). The vein is relatively superficial, covered only by a thin sheet of muscle (platysma), fascia and skin.

### External jugular cannulation

Cannulation of the external jugular vein is relatively easy:

- A slight head-down tilt (15°) will help to distend the vein.

- Distend the vein by occluding it proximally with a finger, just above the clavicle.

- A Seldinger technique may be more successful than using a cannula-over-needle technique.

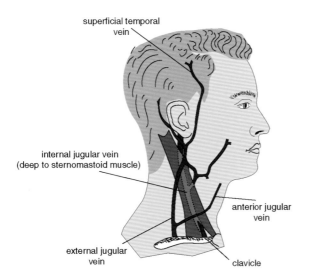

**Figure 9.2 Anatomy of the right external jugular vein**

### Femoral vein

The femoral vein is located just medial to the femoral artery. During cardiac arrest, the absence of a femoral pulse makes localisation of the vein difficult and there is significant risk of accidental arterial injection of drugs.

### Complications

There are several complications of percutaneous venous cannulation; most are relatively minor.

### Early complications

- Failed cannulation: it is best to start distally in a limb and work proximally - if further attempts are required, fluid or drugs will not leak from previous puncture sites.

- Haematoma: secondary to failed cannulation.

- Extravasation of fluid or drugs: the extent of the injury will depend primarily upon the nature of the extravasated fluid.

- Damage to other local structures.

- Air embolus: occurs when the pressure in the veins is lower than in the right side of the heart and air is entrained, or if air is accidentally injected. It is much more likely to occur following cannulation of the external jugular or central veins.

- Shearing of the cannula: this allows fragments to enter the circulation and is caused by trying to reinsert the needle after it has been withdrawn; it is safer to withdraw the whole cannula and attempt cannulation at another site.

### Late complications

- Inflammation of the vein (thrombophlebitis): related to duration of use and the nature of fluids or drugs infused; high concentrations of drugs, fluids with extremes of pH or high osmolality are the main cause.

- Inflammation of the surrounding skin (cellulitis): usually secondary to poor initial aseptic technique, prolonged use, or leakage from the vein.

## Access via the central veins

If venous collapse makes peripheral cannulation difficult access to a central vein may be easier; furthermore, drugs injected into a central vein reach the heart rapidly. However, central veins are deeper than peripheral veins and are often adjacent to major arteries, nerves and other vital structures. Central venous cannulation requires more training and practice than peripheral cannulation, and it usually requires resuscitation to be interrupted. Consequently, the techniques described below are not recommended for inexperienced operators. In the absence of central venous access, a large peripheral vein is perfectly acceptable.

The central veins used most often are the internal jugular vein and the subclavian vein. Recently, the National Institute for Clinical Excellence (NICE) has recommended the use of ultrasound to assist in central venous cannulation. This is unlikely to be practical during cardiopulmonary resuscitation but may be useful when used by an experienced operator attempting central venous cannulation after a spontaneous circulation has been restored.

## Anatomy of the central veins

### The internal jugular vein (Figure 9.3):

- Is lateral to the common carotid artery in the neck.

- Passes beneath the triangle formed by the sternal and clavicular heads of the sternomastoid muscle.

- Joins the subclavian vein, posterior to the sternoclavicular junction to form the brachiocephalic vein.

- The IX-XII cranial nerves and the phrenic nerve are adjacent to the internal jugular vein in the neck.

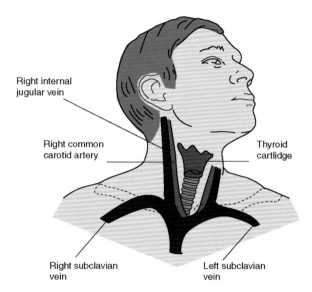

**Figure 9.3 Anatomy of the internal jugular and subclavian veins**

### The subclavian vein (Figure 9.3):

Lies posterior to the medial third of the clavicle and anterior to the subclavian artery; it terminates by joining with the internal jugular vein.

## Equipment

A basic catheter-over-needle device, longer than that used for peripheral intravenous cannulation, can be inserted into a central vein; however, a Seldinger technique is used more commonly:

- Insert a thin-walled, small-diameter needle into the chosen vein. Confirm insertion by free aspiration of blood into the syringe.

- Remove the syringe, insert a guidewire and remove the needle.

- Incise the skin with a scalpel, taking care not to sever the wire.

- Pass a dilator over the wire into the vein.

- Remove the dilator and pass the catheter over the wire into the vein.

- Remove the wire carefully without displacing the catheter.

Single, or multi-lumen 15 cm catheters, 14-16 G, enable monitoring of the central venous pressure and infusion of drugs. Short 7.5-8.5 FG pulmonary artery introducer catheters are ideal for rapid fluid infusion.

## Technique

There are numerous approaches to the internal jugular and subclavian veins. The following is a brief summary only. Whichever vein is chosen:

- use an aseptic technique; if this is not achievable, at least wear sterile gloves;

- dispose of all sharps carefully;

- position the patient 10-15° head down to distend the vein.

### The internal jugular vein

- Turn the patient's head slightly away from the side to be punctured.

- Identify the site of insertion at the apex of the triangle formed by the two heads of the sternomastoid muscle.

- If possible, palpate the carotid artery medial to the puncture site.

- The vein is fairly superficial (1-2 cm deep) and is punctured by aiming the needle slightly laterally and caudally (towards the nipple in the male) (Figure 9.4).

Alternatively, the vein may be punctured by the 'low approach'. The advantages of this technique are that it does not rely on identification of the sternomastoid muscle or the carotid artery, which may be difficult to feel during cardiac arrest.

- Extend the neck slightly and turn the patient's head slightly away from the side of the vein to be punctured. Placement of a bag of fluid or rolled-up towel under the patient's shoulder on the same side will help to extend the neck.

- Palpate the notch on the superior surface of the medial end of the clavicle.

- Insert the needle just above the notch at an angle of 30-40° to the coronal plane.

- Advance the needle posteriorly and caudally; the vein is located at a depth of 1.5-4 cm.

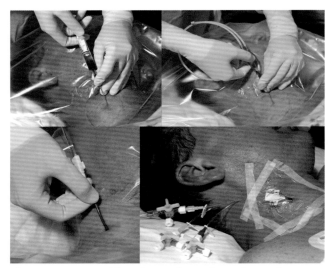

**Figure 9.4 Internal jugular catheter insertion using Seldinger technique**

### The subclavian vein

- Place a bag of fluid or rolled-up towel under the patient's shoulder on the same side as the vein to be punctured and turn the head away slightly.

- Identify the junction of the middle and medial thirds of the clavicle and the suprasternal notch.

- Introduce the needle 1 cm below the junction of the middle and medial thirds of the clavicle, aiming slightly cephalad under the clavicle for the suprasternal notch.

- The vein is usually located when the needle has been inserted 4-6 cm.

### Complications of central venous catheterisation

#### Early complications

- Arterial puncture.

- Haematoma.

- Haemothorax: may occur if the subclavian artery is punctured.

- Pneumothorax: occurs most commonly after using the subclavian approach, or a low approach to the internal jugular vein. In a patient with a pre-existing pneumothorax, it is sensible to attempt to catheterise the subclavian vein on the same side to avoid the risk of creating bilateral pneumothoraces.

- Venous air embolism: this may be caused by a disconnection or a three way tap attached to the catheter being left partly open.

- Cardiac arrhythmias: caused by the guidewire or catheter touching the myocardium. Whenever possible, monitor the ECG during central venous catheterisation.

- The thoracic duct may be lacerated, causing a chylothorax (more common on the left). This is unlikely to become apparent until much later.

- Nerve damage: to the cervical and brachial plexuses.

- Loss of the guidewire into the circulation.

#### Late complications

- Air embolism

- Sepsis

## The intraosseous route for drug delivery

If intravenous access is difficult or impossible, consider the intraosseous route. Although normally considered as an alternative route for vascular access in children, it can also be effective in adults, although the volume of fluid that can be given in this way is unlikely to be effective for volume resuscitation. Intraosseous injection of drugs achieves adequate plasma concentrations in a time comparable to injection through a central venous catheter. The intraosseous route also enables withdrawal of marrow for measurement of electrolytes, glucose and haemoglobin concentration. The intraosseous route for drug delivery will achieve effective plasma concentrations more reliably than the tracheal route.

In adults, the best sites for intraosseous access are the proximal tibia (2 cm below the tibial tuberosity on the antero-medial side) and the distal tibia (2 cm proximal to the medial malleolus). Several intraosseous infusion devices are available (Figure 9.5).

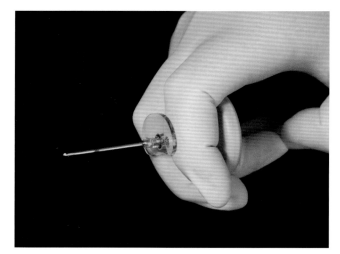

**Figure 9.5 Intraosseus needle**

## The tracheal route for drug delivery

Peripheral venous access may be very difficult, for example, in patients who are profoundly hypovolaemic, hypothermic or are intravenous drug abusers. These factors, combined with lack of operator experience, may preclude central venous cannulation. If intravenous and intraosseous access cannot be established, the tracheal route can be used to give some drugs. Adrenaline, atropine, lidocaine, and naloxone can all be given via the trachea. However, unpredictable plasma concentrations are achieved when drugs are given via a tracheal tube and the optimal tracheal dose of most drugs is unknown. During CPR, studies have shown that the equipotent dose of adrenaline given via the trachea is very variable but is usually 3-10 times higher than the intravenous dose. Calcium salts, sodium bicarbonate, and amiodarone must not be inserted into the trachea.

To achieve plasma concentrations in the therapeutic range, the tracheal dose is at least 3 times the intravenous dose (e.g., adrenaline 3 mg). Inject the drug in a volume of 10-20 ml into the tracheal tube. There is no need to attempt deep bronchial delivery – this does not increase plasma drug concentration any more than tracheal delivery. The solutions in prefilled syringes are acceptable for this purpose although dilution of the drug with water instead of 0.9% saline may achieve better absorption. Giving drugs via a laryngeal mask airway is unreliable because most of the drug is deposited on the larynx; therefore, this route is not recommended.

## Key learning points

- A cannula can be inserted into a peripheral or a central vein.

- The peripheral route is perfectly acceptable initially if a cannula is in place and functioning.

- A central vein enables drugs to be delivered to the central circulation more quickly than a peripheral vein, but central venous cannulation requires specialist skills and equipment.

- Occasionally, venous cannulation will be impossible and the intraosseous or tracheal route, with appropriate adjustment of drug dosage, should be considered.

- The intraosseous route is considerably more reliable than the tracheal route.

## Further reading

International Liaison Committee on Resuscitation. 2005 International Consensus on Cardiopulmonary Resuscitation and Emergency Cardiovascular Care Science with Treatment Recommendations. Part 4. Advanced Life Support. Resuscitation 2005;67:213-47.

Nolan JP, Deakin CD, Soar J, Böttiger BW, Smith G. European Resuscitation Council Guidelines for Resuscitation 2005. Section 4: Adult advanced life support. Resuscitation 2005; 67 Suppl 1:S39-86.

ALS

# Drugs

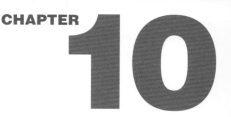

## CHAPTER 10

## Objectives

To understand:

▶ **The indications, doses and actions of the primary drugs used in the treatment of a cardiac arrest.**

▶ **To consider any special precautions or contraindications to the use of these drugs.**

▶ **The indications, doses and actions of drugs used in the peri-arrest period.**

## Introduction

This chapter is divided into two sections:

Section 1: Drugs used during the treatment of a cardiac arrest.

Section 2: Drugs used in the peri-arrest period.

Every effort has been made to provide accurate information on the drugs in this chapter but current publications (e.g., British National Formulary) and current literature from the relevant pharmaceutical companies will provide the most up to date data.

Use prefilled syringes whenever possible for speed and ease of use.

The ALS provider should have a good knowledge of the drugs in Section 1 and should be familiar with the drugs in Section 2.

## Section 1: Drugs used in the treatment of cardiac arrest

Only a few drugs are indicated during the immediate management of a cardiac arrest, and there is only limited scientific evidence supporting their use. Drugs should be considered only after chest compressions and ventilation have been started and, where indicated, defibrillation attempted.

## Oxygen

When available, give high-concentration oxygen to all patients in cardiac arrest. In spontaneously breathing patients give high-concentration oxygen using a mask with an oxygen reservoir. Ensure that the oxygen flow is sufficient (usually > 10 l min⁻¹) to prevent collapse of the reservoir during inspiration. If the patient's trachea is intubated, give high concentration oxygen with a self-inflating bag.

Aim to maintain the $PaO_2$ as close to normal as possible (approximately 13 kPa or 100 mmHg) or 97-100% oxygen saturation on pulse oximetry ($SpO_2$). In some patients this is not possible so you may have to tolerate lower values, i.e., at least <u>above</u> 8 kPa (60 mmHg) or $SpO_2$ 90-92%. In a subgroup of patients with chronic obstructive pulmonary disease (COPD), high concentrations of oxygen may depress breathing. Nevertheless, these patients will also sustain end-organ damage or cardiac arrest if their blood oxygen tensions are allowed to decrease. In this group, aim for a lower than normal $PaO_2$ and oxygen saturation. A suitable target is a $PaO_2$ of 8 kPa (60 mmHg) or 90-92% saturation ($SpO_2$) on pulse oximetry.

## Adrenaline

| Indications | Dose |
|---|---|
| Cardiac arrest of any aetiology | 1 mg IV/IO every 3-5 min |

### Use

Adrenaline is available most commonly in two dilutions:

- 1 in 10,000 (10 ml of this solution contains 1 mg of adrenaline).

- 1 in 1,000 (1 ml of this solution contains 1 mg of adrenaline).

During cardiac arrest, if intravascular (intravenous or intra-osseous) access is delayed or cannot be achieved, give 3 mg, diluted to 10-20 ml with sterile water, via the tracheal tube. Absorption via the tracheal route is highly variable and unreliable.

There is no evidence supporting the use of higher doses of adrenaline for patients in refractory cardiac arrest. In some cases, an adrenaline infusion is required in the post-resuscitation period.

Following return of spontaneous circulation (ROSC), excessive doses of adrenaline may induce tachycardia, myocardial ischaemia, ventricular tachycardia (VT) and ventricular fibrillation (VF). Once a perfusing rhythm is established, if further adrenaline is considered necessary, titrate the dose carefully to achieve an appropriate blood pressure. Intravenous doses of 50-100 mcg are usually sufficient for most hypotensive patients.

### Actions

Adrenaline is a direct-acting sympathomimetic amine that possesses both alpha ($\alpha$) - and beta ($\beta$) -adrenergic activity. In the dose used in resuscitation, adrenaline stimulates both $\alpha_1$- and $\alpha_2$-receptors to produce peripheral vasoconstriction. This increases systemic vascular resistance during CPR, resulting in a relative increase in cerebral and coronary perfusion.

In the beating heart, the action of adrenaline on $\beta_1$ receptors increases heart rate and force of contraction. This is potentially harmful because myocardial oxygen requirement is increased, which may increase ischaemia. The beta-adrenergic effect may enhance cerebral blood flow and is independent of the alpha-mediated increase in perfusion pressure.

Adrenaline increases myocardial excitability and is therefore potentially arrhythmogenic, especially when the myocardium is ischaemic and/or hypoxic. After resuscitation, adrenaline may induce a recurrence of VF.

## Vasopressin

Adrenaline has been the primary sympathomimetic drug in the treatment of cardiac arrest for 40 years. Its primary efficacy is produced by $\alpha$-adrenergic vasoconstrictive effects causing systemic vasoconstriction, which increases coronary and cerebral perfusion pressures. The beta-adrenergic actions of adrenaline (inotropic, chronotropic) may increase coronary and cerebral blood flow, but concomitant increases in myocardial oxygen consumption, ectopic ventricular arrhythmias (particularly when the myocardium is acidotic), and transient hypoxaemia caused by pulmonary arteriovenous shunting may offset these benefits.

The potentially deleterious beta effects of adrenaline have led to a search for alternative vasopressors. Vasopressin is a naturally occurring anti-diuretic hormone. In very high doses it is a powerful vasoconstrictor that acts by stimulation of smooth muscle V1 receptors. The importance of vasopressin in cardiac arrest was first recognised in studies of out-of-hospital cardiac arrest patients when vasopressin concentrations were found to be higher in successfully resuscitated patients. Although clinical and animal studies show improved haemodynamic values when using vasopressin as an alternative to adrenaline during resuscitation from cardiac arrest, not all have shown improved survival.

Two large, randomised studies have compared vasopressin with adrenaline for in-hospital and out-of-hospital cardiac arrest. In both studies patients were randomised to receive vasopressin or adrenaline initially and those refractory to the initial drug were given adrenaline as rescue treatment. Both studies were unable to demonstrate an overall increase in the rates of ROSC or survival for vasopressin 40 U, with the dose repeated in one study, when compared with adrenaline (1 mg, repeated), as the initial vasopressor. In the large out-of-hospital cardiac arrest study, post-hoc analysis (i.e., not planned before the study started) suggested that the subset of patients with asystole had significant improvement in survival to discharge but there was no difference in the numbers who survived neurologically intact.

A recent meta-analysis of five randomised trials showed no statistically significant difference between vasopressin and adrenaline for ROSC, death within 24 h, or death before hospital discharge. The sub-group analysis based on initial cardiac rhythm did not show any statistically significant difference in the rate of death before hospital discharge.

There is currently insufficient evidence to support or refute the use of vasopressin as an alternative to, or in combination with, adrenaline in any cardiac arrest rhythm. Current practice supports continued use of adrenaline as the primary vasopressor for the treatment of cardiac arrest of all rhythms.

## Amiodarone

| Indications | Dose |
|---|---|
| Refractory ventricular fibrillation/ pulseless VT (VF/VT) | 300 mg IV |

### Use

Amiodarone may paradoxically be arrhythmogenic, especially if given concurrently with drugs that prolong the QT interval. But, it has a lower incidence of pro-arrhythmic effects than other antiarrhythmic drugs under similar circumstances.

The major, acute adverse effects from amiodarone are hypotension and bradycardia, which will not be apparent until after a spontaneous circulation has been restored. The side effects associated with prolonged oral use (photosensitivity, abnormalities of thyroid function, peripheral neuropathy, pulmonary inflammation/fibrosis and hepatic dysfunction) are not relevant in the acute setting.

Consider an initial intravenous bolus dose of 300 mg amiodarone, diluted in 5% dextrose to 20 ml (or from a prefilled syringe), if VF/VT persists after the third shock. Amiodarone can cause thrombophlebitis when injected into a peripheral vein: use a central vein if the patient already has a central venous catheter in situ; if not, use a large peripheral vein and a generous flush. Details about the use of amiodarone for the treatment of other arrhythmias are given in Section 2.

Following three initial stacked shocks, in shock refractory VF amiodarone improves the short-term outcome of survival to hospital admission compared with placebo or lidocaine. Amiodarone also appears to improve the response to defibrillation when given to humans or animals with VF or haemodynamically unstable ventricular tachycardia.

There is no evidence to indicate the time at which amiodarone should be given when using a single-shock strategy. In the clinical studies to date, the amiodarone was given if VF/VT persisted after at least three shocks. For this reason, and in the absence of any other data, amiodarone 300 mg is recommended if VF/VT persists after 3 shocks.

## Actions

Amiodarone is a membrane stabilising antiarrhythmic drug that increases the duration of the action potential and refractory period in atrial and ventricular myocardium.

Atrioventricular conduction is slowed, and there is a similar effect on accessory pathways. Amiodarone has a very mild negative inotropic action and causes some peripheral vasodilation by non-competitive α-blockade. The hypotension caused by intravenous amiodarone is worse with rapid injection and is caused more by the solvent (Polysorbate 80), which causes histamine release, rather than the drug itself. The use of an aqueous amiodarone preparation that is relatively free from these side effects is encouraged but is not yet widely available.

# Lidocaine

| Indications | Dose |
| --- | --- |
| Refractory ventricular fibrillation/pulseless VT (when amiodarone is unavailable) | 100 mg IV |

## Use

Consider lidocaine 100 mg (1-1.5 mg kg$^{-1}$) for the treatment of VF/VT refractory to three shocks, but only when amiodarone is unavailable. Give an additional bolus of 50 mg if necessary. Do not exceed 3 mg kg$^{-1}$ during the first hour. Comparative studies indicate that amiodarone is a better antiarrhythmic drug than lidocaine.

Lidocaine is metabolised by the liver and its half-life is prolonged if hepatic blood flow is reduced, e.g., in the presence of reduced cardiac output, liver disease or in the elderly. During cardiac arrest, normal clearance mechanisms do not function and high plasma concentrations may be achieved after a single dose. After 24 h of continuous infusion the plasma half-life increases significantly. Give reduced doses in these circumstances and review regularly the indication for continued therapy. Lidocaine is less effective in the presence of hypokalaemia and hypomagnesaemia, which should be corrected immediately.

## Actions

Lidocaine is a membrane stabilising antiarrhythmic drug that acts by increasing the myocyte refractory period. It decreases ventricular automaticity and ectopic activity. Lidocaine suppresses activity of depolarised, arrhythmogenic tissues while interfering minimally with the electrical activity of normal tissues. Therefore, it is effective in suppressing arrhythmias associated with depolarisation (e.g., ischaemia, digitalis toxicity) but is relatively ineffective against arrhythmias occurring in normally polarised cells (e.g., atrial fibrillation/flutter). Lidocaine increases the threshold for VF.

An excessive dose of lidocaine (> 3 mg kg$^{-1}$ over the first hour) can cause paraesthesia, drowsiness, confusion, and muscular twitching progressing to convulsions. If there are signs of toxicity, stop the infusion immediately; treat seizures if they occur. Lidocaine depresses myocardial function, but this is usually transient and can be treated with intravenous fluids or vasopressors.

# Magnesium Sulphate

| Indications | Dose |
| --- | --- |
| Shock refractory ventricular fibrillation in the presence of hypomagnesaemia | 2 g bolus IV |
| Ventricular tachyarrhythmias in the presence of hypomagnesaemia | 2 g over 10 min IV |
| Torsade de pointes | |
| Atrial fibrillation | |
| Digoxin toxicity | |

## Use

Intravenous magnesium is safe and often effective treatment for ventricular tachyarrhythmias. Magnesium is excreted by the kidneys but side effects associated with hypermagnesaemia are rare, even in renal failure. Magnesium inhibits smooth muscle contraction, leading to vasodilation, causing flushing (in conscious patients) and dose-related hypotension; this is usually transient and responds to intravenous fluids and vasopressors.

In shock-refractory VF, give an initial intravenous bolus dose of 2 g (= 4 ml (8 mmol)) of 50% magnesium sulphate; it may be repeated after 10-15 min. For other tachyarrhythmias (table above) give 2 g over 10 min.

## Actions

Magnesium is an important constituent of many enzyme systems, especially those involved with ATP generation in muscle. It plays a major role in neurochemical transmission where it decreases acetylcholine release and reduces the sensitivity of the motor end plate. Magnesium also improves the contractile response of the stunned myocardium and limits infarct size by an as yet unknown mechanism. The normal plasma concentration of magnesium is 0.80–1.00 mmol l$^{-1}$.

Magnesium deficiency is not uncommon in hospitalised patients and frequently co-exists with other electrolyte disturbances, particularly hypokalaemia, hypophosphataemia, hyponatraemia and hypocalcaemia. Hypomagnesaemia may contribute to arrhythmias and cardiac arrest. Hypomagnesaemia increases myocardial digoxin uptake and decreases cellular Na+/K$^+$-ATPase activity. Patients with hypomagnesaemia, hypokalaemia, or both may develop cardiac manifestations of digoxin toxicity, even with plasma concentrations of digoxin in the quoted therapeutic range.

ALS

Although the benefits of giving magnesium in known hypomagnesaemic states are recognised, giving magnesium routinely during cardiac arrest has not proven to be of benefit. Studies in adults in- and out-of-hospital have failed to demonstrate any increase in the rate of ROSC when magnesium is given routinely during CPR. There is some evidence to suggest that magnesium may be of benefit in refractory VF.

# Other Drugs

As with most drugs used in the treatment of cardiac arrest, the evidence for the benefit of other drugs, including atropine, calcium and sodium bicarbonate, given routinely during human cardiac arrest is limited. The recommendations for their use are based on our understanding of the pathophysiology of cardiac arrest and the pharmacodynamic properties of the drugs

## Atropine

| Indications | Dose |
| --- | --- |
| Asystole | 3 mg IV once only |
| Pulseless electrical activity (PEA) with a heart rate < 60 min$^{-1}$ | |

### Use

There is no conclusive evidence that atropine is of value in asystolic cardiac arrest. However, asystole carries a grave prognosis and there are anecdotal accounts of success after giving atropine. It is unlikely to be harmful in this situation.

The recommended adult dose for asystole or PEA with a rate < 60 min$^{-1}$ is 3 mg intravenously in a single dose. Its use in the treatment of bradycardia is covered in Section 2.

### Actions

Atropine antagonises the action of the parasympathetic neurotransmitter acetylcholine at muscarinic receptors. Therefore it blocks the effect of the vagus nerve on both the sinoatrial (SA) node and the atrioventricular (AV) node, increasing sinus automaticity and facilitating AV node conduction.

Side-effects of atropine are dose-related (blurred vision, dry mouth and urinary retention); they are not relevant during a cardiac arrest. Acute confusional states may occur following intravenous injection, particularly in elderly patients. After cardiac arrest, do not attribute dilated pupils solely to atropine. Several recent studies have failed to demonstrate any benefit from atropine in out-of-hospital or in-hospital cardiac arrests.

## Calcium

| Indications | Dose |
| --- | --- |
| Pulseless electrical activity caused by:<br>• Hyperkalaemia<br>• Hypocalcaemia<br>• Overdose of calcium channel blocking drugs<br>• Hypermagnesaemia | 10 ml 10% calcium chloride IV |

### Use

Calcium can slow the heart rate and precipitate arrhythmias. In cardiac arrest, calcium may be given by rapid intravenous injection. In the presence of a spontaneous circulation, give it slowly. Calcium solutions and sodium bicarbonate should not be given simultaneously by the same route.

The initial dose of 10 ml 10% calcium chloride (6.8 mmol Ca$^{2+}$) may be repeated if necessary.

### Actions

Calcium plays a vital role in the cellular mechanisms underlying myocardial contraction. There are few data supporting any beneficial action for calcium following most cases of cardiac arrest. High plasma concentrations achieved after injection may have detrimental effects on the ischaemic myocardium and may impair cerebral recovery. Thus, calcium is given during resuscitation only when specifically indicated.

## Sodium bicarbonate

| Indications | Dose |
| --- | --- |
| Life-threatening hyperkalaemia or cardiac arrest associated with hyperkalaemia | 50 ml 8.4% sodium bicarbonate IV |
| Tricyclic overdose | |

### Use

Giving sodium bicarbonate routinely during cardiac arrest and CPR (especially in out-of-hospital cardiac arrests) or after ROSC is not recommended. Give sodium bicarbonate (50 mmol) if cardiac arrest is associated with hyperkalaemia or tricyclic antidepressant overdose; repeat the dose according to the clinical condition and result of repeated blood gas analysis. Some experts give bicarbonate if the arterial pH is less than 7.1, but this is controversial. During cardiac arrest, arterial blood gas values do not reflect the acid base state of the tissues - the tissue pH will be lower than that in arterial blood. Mixed venous blood values give a more accurate estimate of the pH in the tissues, but it is rare for a pulmonary artery catheter to be in situ at the time of cardiac arrest. If a central venous catheter is in situ, central venous blood gas analysis will provide a closer estimate of tissue acid base state than that provided by arterial blood.

## Actions

Giving bicarbonate causes generation of carbon dioxide, which diffuses rapidly into cells: this exacerbates intracellular acidosis and has a negative inotropic effect on ischaemic myocardium. Injection of bicarbonate presents a large, osmotically active sodium load to an already compromised circulation and brain. It shifts the oxygen dissociation curve to the left, further inhibiting release of oxygen to the tissues.

Mild acidosis causes vasodilation and can increase cerebral blood flow. Therefore, full correction of the arterial blood pH may theoretically reduce cerebral blood flow at a particularly critical time. As the bicarbonate ion is excreted as carbon dioxide via the lungs, ventilation needs to be increased. For all these reasons metabolic acidaemia must be severe to justify giving sodium bicarbonate.

## Fluids

Hypovolaemia is a potentially reversible cause of cardiac arrest – infuse fluids if hypovolaemia is suspected. In the initial stages of resuscitation, there are no clear advantages to using colloid. Use 0.9% saline or Hartmann's solution. Avoid dextrose – this will be redistributed rapidly away from the intravascular space and will cause hyperglycaemia, which may worsen neurological outcome after cardiac arrest. In cases of hypovolaemia where the cause is surgically remediable (e.g., post- operative, ruptured aortic aneurysm, trauma), slow the fluid infusion once a radial pulse is palpable. Consider immediate surgery at this stage. Excessive fluid infusion can exacerbate bleeding and cause dilution of vital clotting factors.

Whether fluids should be infused routinely during cardiac arrest is controversial. There are no published human studies of routine fluid use compared to no fluids during normovolaemic cardiac arrest. In the absence of hypovolaemia, infusion of an excessive volume of fluid during CPR is likely to be harmful. Use intravenous fluid to flush peripherally injected drugs into the central circulation. If ROSC is achieved, fluid infusion may be indicated based on clinical assessment and haemodynamic values.

## Thrombolytic therapy during CPR

| Indications | Dose |
| --- | --- |
| Cardiac arrest caused by suspected pulmonary embolus | • Tenecteplase 500-600 mcg kg$^{-1}$ IV over 10 sec<br>• Alteplase (r-tPA) 10 mg IV over 1-2 min followed by IV infusion of 90 mg over 2 h |

### Use

Following thrombolytic therapy given during CPR for acute pulmonary embolism, survival and good neurological outcome has been reported even in patients requiring more than 60 min CPR. If a thrombolytic drug is given in these circumstances, consider continuing CPR for at least 60-90 min before termination of resuscitation attempts.

### Indications

Consider thrombolytic therapy when cardiac arrest is caused by proven or suspected acute pulmonary embolus. There are currently insufficient clinical data to recommend the routine use of thrombolytic therapy during non-traumatic cardiac arrest. Attempted thrombolysis may be considered in adult cardiac arrest on a case-by-case basis following initial failure of standard resuscitation in patients in whom an acute thrombotic aetiology for the arrest is suspected. Ongoing CPR is not a contraindication to thrombolytic therapy.

### Actions

Adult cardiac arrest is caused usually by acute myocardial ischaemia following coronary artery occlusion by thrombus. There are several reports on the successful use of thrombolytic therapy during cardiac arrest, particularly when the arrest was caused by pulmonary embolism. The use of thrombolytic drugs to break down coronary artery and pulmonary artery thrombus has been the subject of several studies. In animal studies, thrombolytic drugs have beneficial effects on cerebral blood flow during cardiopulmonary resuscitation and a clinical study has reported less hypoxic encephalopathy after thrombolytic therapy during CPR.

Several studies have examined the use of thrombolytic therapy given during non-traumatic cardiac arrest refractory to standard therapy. Two studies have shown an increase in ROSC with non-significant improvements in survival to hospital discharge and a further study demonstrated greater ICU survival.

When given to cardiac arrest patients with suspected or proven pulmonary embolus, two studies have shown possible benefits, one finding an improvement in 24-h survival. Several clinical studies and case series have not demonstrated any increase in bleeding complications of thrombolytic therapy during CPR in non-traumatic cardiac arrest.

ALS

## Section 2. Drugs used in the peri-arrest period

This section provides detailed information on the drugs used in the peri-arrest period. The role of atropine, amiodarone, and lidocaine in the treatment of cardiac arrest has been considered in Section 1. The drugs are listed in alphabetical order.

Remember that drugs that can treat arrhythmias can also cause arrhythmias.

## Adenosine

| Indications | Dose |
|---|---|
| Stable regular narrow-complex tachycardia (or broad-complex tachycardia known to be an supraventricular tachycardia (SVT) with bundle branch block) that is not terminated by vagal manoeuvres. | 6 mg, 12 mg, 12 mg IV |

### Use

Give adenosine in a monitored environment only (e.g., cardiac care unit, critical care unit, operating room, or emergency department); it may cause a transient period of ventricular standstill.

The major advantage of adenosine is that, unlike verapamil, it can be given to a patient with a broad-complex tachycardia of uncertain aetiology. The ventricular rate in SVT will be slowed transiently but ventricular tachycardia (VT) will continue unchanged. Adenosine is effective in terminating the vast majority of tachycardias that are caused by a re-entry circuit that passes through the AV node. Another advantage is that adenosine does not cause significant negative inotropic effects so does not cause decreased cardiac output and hypotension. Adenosine can be given safely to a patient who is taking a beta-blocker.

Warn patients of transient unpleasant side-effects, in particular nausea, flushing, and chest discomfort. Adenosine is not available in some European countries, but adenosine triphosphate (ATP) is an alternative. In a few European countries neither preparation may be available; verapamil is probably the next best choice.

Theophylline and related compounds block the effect of adenosine. Patients taking dipyridamole or carbamazepine, or with denervated hearts display a markedly exaggerated effect that may be hazardous. In the presence of Wolff-Parkinson-White (WPW) syndrome, blockade of conduction through the AV node by adenosine may promote conduction down an accessory pathway. In the presence of pre-excited atrial fibrillation or flutter this may cause a dangerously rapid ventricular response.

The smallest dose likely to be effective is 6 mg (which is outside some current licenses for an initial dose); if

unsuccessful follow this with up to two doses each of 12 mg at intervals of 1-2 min.

### Action

Adenosine is a naturally occurring purine nucleotide. It slows transmission across the AV node but has little effect on other myocardial cells or conduction pathways. It is highly effective for terminating paroxysmal SVT with re-entrant circuits that include the AV node (AVNRT and AVRT). In other narrow-complex tachycardias (e.g., atrial flutter) adenosine will reveal the underlying atrial rhythm by slowing the ventricular response. It has an extremely short half-life of 10-15 sec and, therefore, is given as a rapid bolus into a fast running intravenous infusion or followed by a 0.9% saline flush.

## Amiodarone

| Indications | Dose |
|---|---|
| Control of haemodynamically stable VT, polymorphic VT, and broad-complex tachycardia of uncertain origin | 300 mg IV over 20-60 min followed by an infusion of 900 mg over 24 h |
| Paroxysmal SVT uncontrolled by adenosine, vagal manoeuvres, and AV nodal blockade | |
| To control rapid ventricular rate caused by accessory pathway conduction in pre-excited atrial arrhythmias | |
| Haemodynamically unstable tachycardia unresponsive to attempted electrical cardioversion. | 300 mg IV over 10-20 min followed by an infusion of 900 mg over 24 h. |

### Use

Give amiodarone 300 mg intravenously over 10-60 min depending on the circumstances and haemodynamic stability of the patient. This loading dose is followed by an infusion of 900 mg over 24 h. Give additional doses of 150 mg as necessary for recurrent or resistant arrhythmias to a maximum total daily dose of 2 g (the maximum licensed dose varies between different countries). In patients known to have severely impaired heart function, intravenous amiodarone is preferable to other antiarrhythmic drugs for atrial and ventricular arrhythmias. Major adverse effects from amiodarone are hypotension and bradycardia, which can be prevented by slowing the rate of drug infusion. Whenever possible, give intravenous amiodarone via a central venous catheter – it causes thrombophlebitis when infused into a peripheral vein. In an emergency it can be injected into a large peripheral vein.

The plasma levels of warfarin and digoxin are increased by amiodarone; therefore their doses should be reduced. The dose of warfarin usually requires reduction by one third and digoxin by half; monitor the INR for warfarin and digoxin levels to guide digoxin therapy. Amiodarone has an additive effect to that of beta-blockers and calcium channel blockers on the degree of AV nodal blockade.

## Aspirin

| Indications | Dose |
|---|---|
| • Acute coronary syndromes (Chapter 3) | 300-325 mg oral loading dose followed by 75 mg daily |

### Use

Give aspirin orally in a single dose of 300-325 mg. Aspirin efficacy seems to be similar in patients treated early or late; give aspirin to patients with acute coronary syndromes (Chapter 3) irrespective of the delay to the first evaluation of the patient. Regular use of aspirin can cause acute or chronic upper gastro-intestinal bleeding. The risk is dose-related.

Since the anti-platelet activity of aspirin may be achieved within 30 min, do not delay giving aspirin until arrival in hospital, unless contraindications are recognised. Aspirin is simple to give and a single dose is well tolerated.

If thrombolytic therapy is given in the early phase, give aspirin concomitantly to help reduce the risk of early coronary artery reocclusion.

### Actions

Aspirin improves the prognosis of patients with acute coronary syndromes, significantly reducing cardiovascular death. The efficacy of aspirin is achieved by anti-platelet activity and anti-thrombotic protection.

## Atropine

| Indications | Dose |
|---|---|
| Sinus, atrial, or nodal bradycardia when the patient displays adverse signs | 500 mcg increments IV to a maximum of 3 mg |

### Use

Give an initial dose of 0.5-1 mg IV. Repeated doses may be necessary subsequently, but consider pacing if this is ineffective (Chapter 11).

Conduction disturbance or bradycardia associated with high vagal tone may respond to atropine.

## Beta-adrenergic blockers

| Indications | Dose |
|---|---|
| • Narrow-complex regular tachycardias uncontrolled by vagal manoeuvres and adenosine in the patient with preserved ventricular function<br>• To control rate in AF and atrial flutter when the duration of arrhythmia is less than 48 h and ventricular function is preserved | • Atenolol ($\beta_1$) 5 mg IV over 5 min<br>• Metoprolol ($\beta_1$) 2-5 mg IV at 5 min intervals to total dose of 15 mg<br>• Propanolol ($\beta_1$ and $\beta_2$) 100 mcg kg$^{-1}$ in 3 divided doses at 2 min intervals<br>• Esmolol ($\beta_1$) 500 mcg kg$^{-1}$ over 1 min followed by an infusion of 50-200 mcg kg$^{-1}$ min$^{-1}$ |

### Use

A beta-blocker is a second-line drug for the treatment of narrow-complex tachycardia (or broad complex tachycardia known to be an SVT with aberrant conduction), after the use of adenosine (Chapter 12). The use of any beta-blocker may precipitate left ventricular failure in patients with a failing ventricle, hypotension, or heart block. Profound bradycardia may develop and may be difficult to treat. The risk of heart block or asystole is increased if verapamil is given intravenously to a beta-blocked patient, especially if the beta-blocker is also given intravenously. For similar reasons, avoid the combination of beta-blockers and other antiarrhythmic drugs such as lidocaine.

When treating SVT, be careful to avoid converting a non-life-threatening condition into one that is life-threatening by injudicious use of multiple drugs.

IV esmolol is a short-acting (half-life of 2-9 min) $\beta_1$-selective beta-blocker.

### Actions

Beta-blocking drugs (atenolol, metoprolol, labetalol (alpha- and beta-blocking effects), propranolol, esmolol) reduce the effects of circulating catecholamines and decrease heart rate and blood pressure. They also have cardioprotective effects in patients with acute coronary syndromes.

Side effects of beta-blockade include bradycardia, AV conduction delay, hypotension and bronchospasm. Contraindications to the use of beta-blocking drugs include second- or third-degree heart block, hypotension, severe congestive heart failure, and lung disease associated with bronchospasm.

ALS

## Calcium channel blockers: verapamil and diltiazem

| Indications | Dose |
|---|---|
| Stable regular narrow complex tachycardia that is not terminated by vagal manoeuvres or adenosine | Verapamil 2.5–5mg IV over 2 min  or diltiazem 15-20 mg IV over 2 min |
| Control of ventricular rate in patients with AF or atrial flutter (usually when the duration of the arrhythmia is less than 48 h) | Diltiazem 15-20 mg  IV over 2 min |

### Use

Intravenous verapamil is used in the treatment of SVT only when the diagnosis has been established firmly. It has a significant negative inotropic effect and must not be given to a patient with broad complex tachycardia of ventricular or doubtful origin.

Side effects, in common with other vasodilators, include flushing, headaches and hypotension. The hypotension can be severe; the antiarrhythmic effect persists for about 6 h after an intravenous dose.

The initial dose of verapamil is 2.5-5 mg IV given over 2 min. In the absence of a therapeutic response or drug-induced adverse event, give repeated doses of 5-10 mg every 15-30 min to a maximum of 20 mg. Reassess the patient carefully after each dose. Give verapamil only to patients with narrow-complex paroxysmal SVT or arrhythmia known with certainty to be of supraventricular origin.

Diltiazem 0.25 mg kg$^{-1}$, followed by a second dose of 0.35 mg kg$^{-1}$, is as effective as verapamil. Intravenous diltiazem is not available in some countries (e.g., UK). Verapamil, and to a lesser extent, diltiazem may decrease myocardial contractility and critically reduce cardiac output in patients with severe left ventricular dysfunction. For the reason stated under adenosine (above), calcium channel blockers may be harmful when given to patients with pre-excited AF or atrial flutter associated with WPW syndrome.

### Actions

Verapamil and diltiazem are calcium channel blocking drugs that slow conduction and increase refractoriness in the AV node. These actions may terminate re-entry arrhythmia that involves the AV node and contribute to control of ventricular response rate in patients with other atrial tachyarrythmias.

## Digoxin

| Indications | Dose |
|---|---|
| Atrial fibrillation with fast ventricular response | 500 mcg IV over 30 min |

### Use

Digoxin has limited use as an antiarrhythmic drug. It can decrease ventricular rate in patients with atrial fibrillation with a rapid ventricular response, but in acute atrial fibrillation is slow in onset and less effective than other antiarrhythmic drugs, such as amiodarone or beta-blockers.

Side effects increase in severity as the serum digoxin concentration rises. They include nausea, diarrhoea, anorexia, confusion and dizziness. Other arrhythmias may also develop as a result of digoxin toxicity. Digoxin toxicity is increased by hypokalaemia, hypomagnesaemia, hypoxia, hypercalcaemia, renal failure, and hypothyroidism.  It can be confirmed by direct measurement of plasma concentrations.

Rapid digitalisation can be achieved intravenously or by a combination of intravenous and oral loading doses. A maximum dose of 500 mcg digoxin in 50 ml 5% dextrose, is given intravenously over 30 min, repeated once if necessary. If the patient is small, old, or frail, use a lower loading dose. The oral maintenance dose is 62.5-500 mcg per day but the risk of toxicity increases greatly with doses above 250 mcg. The half-life of digoxin is approximately 36 h in patients with normal renal function, but will be prolonged substantially in the presence of renal impairment.

### Actions

Digoxin is a cardiac glycoside that slows ventricular rate by:

* increasing vagal tone;

* decreasing sympathetic activity by suppression of baroreceptors;

* prolonging AV node refractory period.

It also enhances myocardial contractility and enhances automaticity and decreases conduction velocity in the Purkinje fibres.

## Inotropes and vasopressors: dobutamine, adrenaline, noradrenaline, and dopamine

### Dobutamine

| Indications | Dose |
|---|---|
| • Hypotension not caused by hypovolaemia<br>• Cardiogenic shock | 5-20 mcg kg$^{-1}$ min$^{-1}$ |

### Use

Dobutamine is often the inotropic drug of choice in the post-resuscitation period. It is indicated when poor cardiac output and hypotension cause significantly reduced tissue perfusion. It is useful particularly when pulmonary oedema is present and hypotension prevents the use of other vasodilators. Haemodynamic monitoring of the patient is essential and should be undertaken in a high-dependency or intensive care area. Try to avoid inducing a tachycardia, which will exacerbate myocardial ischaemia. Cardiac arrhythmias may occur, particularly at higher doses. Reduce the infusion slowly to avoid hypotension.

The drug has a short half-life and is given by intravenous infusion using an infusion pump. The typical dose range is 5-20 mcg $kg^{-1}$ $min^{-1}$ titrated to the response of blood pressure and/or cardiac output.

## Actions

Dobutamine is a synthetic catecholamine with effects mediated by $\beta_1$, $\beta_2$, and $\alpha_1$-receptors. It exerts a positive inotropic action on the myocardium by stimulating $\beta_1$ receptors. In peripheral blood vessels, $\beta_2$-stimulation causes vasodilation, which reduces peripheral resistance and may reduce blood pressure. The net effect is to increase cardiac output. Renal blood flow is usually increased. Dobutamine increases myocardial oxygen requirements less than other inotropic agents and is less likely to cause arrhythmias.

## Adrenaline

| Indications | Dose |
|---|---|
| Second-line treatment for cardiogenic shock. | 0.05–1 mcg $kg^{-1}$ $min^{-1}$ |
| As an alternative to external pacing for bradycardia. | 2–10 mcg $min^{-1}$ |
| Anaphylaxis | See Chapter 13 |

## Use

An adrenaline infusion is indicated in the post-resuscitation period when less potent inotropic drugs (such as dobutamine) have failed to increase cardiac output adequately. It is indicated also for bradycardia associated with adverse signs and or risk of asystole, which has not responded to atropine, if external pacing is unavailable or unsuccessful.

When given by infusion in the post-resuscitation period, the dose is typically 0.05-1 mcg $kg^{-1}$ $min^{-1}$. Start the infusion at a low rate and titrate to the mean arterial pressure and/or cardiac output. When given for atropine-resistant bradycardia the effective dose range is usually 2–10 mcg $min^{-1}$.

## Actions

The alpha- and beta-agonist actions of adrenaline normally cause a substantial increase in contractility and vasoconstriction. This will usually increase blood pressure and cardiac output, but the accompanying tachycardia and increase in afterload may cause substantial myocardial ischaemia. Adrenaline can also cause ischaemia of the gut.

## Noradrenaline

| Indications | Dose |
|---|---|
| • Severe hypotension associated with low peripheral resistance (e.g., septic shock), and in the absence of hypovolaemia<br>• An alternative to adrenaline in the treatment for cardiogenic shock | 0.05-1 mcg $kg^{-1}$ $min^{-1}$ |

## Use

Noradrenaline is indicated in the post resuscitation period when hypotension and poor cardiac output cause significantly reduced tissue perfusion. Correct hypovolaemia first. Noradrenaline is particularly effective when cardiac arrest has occurred in association with profound peripheral vasodilation (e.g., sepsis or other conditions causing the systemic inflammatory response syndrome (SIRS)). It may be used in combination with dobutamine. Haemodynamic monitoring of the patient in a critical care area is essential. Noradrenaline must be given via a central vein: subcutaneous extravasation will cause severe tissue necrosis.

The drug has a short half-life and must be given by intravenous infusion, using an infusion pump. The smallest effective dose should be used, starting at approximately 0.05 mcg $kg^{-1}$ $min^{-1}$ and titrated to the response of arterial pressure.

## Actions

Noradrenaline is a catecholamine with potent agonist effects on alpha-receptors. It also has some agonist effects on beta-receptors. The net result is marked vasoconstriction and some positive inotropic action on the myocardium. Many factors influence the precise effect on cardiac output (blood volume, vascular resistance, etc.), but it is usually increased. Noradrenaline may increase myocardial oxygen demand but this may be offset by increased coronary perfusion pressure and myocardial oxygen delivery.

## Dopamine

| Indications | Dose |
|---|---|
| Hypotension in the absence of hypovolaemia | 1-10 mcg $kg^{-1}$ $min^{-1}$ |

## Use

There is considerable individual variability in the response to dopamine and it is impossible to select a dose to target specific receptors. Dopamine will often increase urine volume but has no beneficial effect on renal function per se. Dopamine should be given via a central vein, using an infusion pump. Use of dopamine requires invasive monitoring in an intensive care or high-dependency care area.

ALS

Dopamine is given as an intravenous infusion at 1-2 mcg kg$^{-1}$ min$^{-1}$ initially. The dose used to increase cardiac output and blood pressure is typically in the range of 5-10 mcg kg$^{-1}$ min$^{-1}$.

## Actions

Dopamine is the precursor of the naturally-occurring catecholamines adrenaline and noradrenaline. It has a dose-dependant positive inotropic effect that is mediated by dopamine ($D_1$ and $D_2$), alpha$_1$-, and beta$_1$- receptors. In theory, low infusion rates (1-2 mcg kg$^{-1}$min$^{-1}$) cause renal artery vasodilation (via $D_1$ receptors), and increase glomerular filtration rate and sodium excretion. In reality, 'low-dose' dopamine may also produce effects mediated by alpha- and beta- receptors. Intermediate infusion rates (2-10 mcg kg$^{-1}$min$^{-1}$) increase cardiac output and systolic blood pressure ($\beta_1$). With highest infusion rates (> 10 mcg kg$^{-1}$ min$^{-1}$) $\alpha_1$- and $\alpha_2$- receptors are activated causing widespread vasoconstriction. Dopamine may cause cardiac arrhythmias, increase myocardial oxygen demand and worsen ischaemia.

## Lidocaine

| Indications | Dose |
|---|---|
| Haemodynamically stable ventricular tachycardia (as an alternative to amiodarone) | 50 mg IV |

## Use

Lidocaine is an alternative to amiodarone for the initial treatment of ventricular tachycardia without adverse signs.

Give lidocaine 50 mg intravenously. This will be distributed rapidly and may be effective for only 10 min. If needed, repeat this dose every 5 min up to a maximum dose of 200 mg.

## Naloxone

| Indications | Dose |
|---|---|
| Opioid overdose (Chapter 13) | 400–800 mcg IV |

## Use

Naloxone will reverse all the effects of exogenous opioids, in particular, cerebral and respiratory depression. The duration of action is very short so that repeated injections are often required. Reversal of the effect of opioids may exacerbate pain or cause restless behaviour in patients dependent on opioids.

Adults may need an initial dose of 400-800 mcg intravenously. Repeat this every 2-3 min, if necessary, up to 10 mg. Alternatively, give an infusion of naloxone titrated to achieve the desired effect.

## Action

Naloxone is a specific competitive antagonist at mu-, delta-, and kappa-opioid receptors.

## Nitrates

| Indications | Dose |
|---|---|
| Prophylaxis or relief of angina | GTN: 300-600 mcg sublingual |
| Unstable angina pectoris | Sublingual 400 mcg, buccal tablets 1-5 mg |
| Myocardial infarction | Buccal 5 mg, transdermal 5-15 mg |
| Acute and chronic left ventricular failure (LVF) | 10-200 mcg min$^{-1}$ IV Isosobide mono- or dinitrate: 10-60 mg oral |

## Use

The duration of action depends on the nitrate preparation used and mode of delivery. Nitrates delivered via the buccal and sublingual routes are effective within 1-2 min. If side effects occur removing the tablet will enable them to settle. Safe use of intravenous nitrates requires haemodynamic monitoring because they can cause significant hypotension. Do not give nitrates to patients who are already significantly hypotensive. Other side effects include flushing and headache.

Glyceryl trinitrate (GTN) may be given by sublingual tablet (300-600 mcg), by metered spray (400 mcg), by buccal absorption (1-5 mg), or by transdermal absorption (5-15 mg) and repeated as required. It may also be given intravenously (10-200 mcg min$^{-1}$). Isosorbide mono- or dinitrate may be given orally (30-120 mg daily total dose).

## Action

After conversion to nitric oxide, nitrates cause vascular smooth muscle relaxation. The resultant dilation is more marked on the venous than the arterial side of the circulation. Thus, myocardial preload is reduced proportionately more than afterload. This improves coronary flow to the sub-endocardial myocardium by lowering diastolic pressure inside the left ventricle. Nitrates also dilate the coronary arteries and relieve spasm in coronary smooth muscle.

## Opioids

| Indications | Dose |
|---|---|
| • Analgesia<br>• Acute left ventricular failure (LVF) | • Morphine 5-20 mg IV<br>• Diamorphine 2.5-10 mg IV |

## Use

Give opioids by slow intravenous injection and titrate the dose to the patient's response. This should prevent the sudden onset of profound respiratory depression, hypotension, or bradycardia. The dose will also depend on

ALS

the age and size of the patient. Respiratory depression or hypotension can be reversed by naloxone. Give anti-emetic drugs concurrently to suppress opioid induced nausea and vomiting.

Adult doses of 2.5-10 mg diamorphine and 5-20 mg morphine are equipotent.

### Action

Morphine and diamorphine (which is not available in many countries) are opioid analgesics. They reduce ventricular preload and afterload by increasing venous capacitance and by mild arterial vasodilation, thereby reducing myocardial oxygen demand.

## Thrombolytic therapy in acute myocardial infarction

### Indications

Presentation within 12 h, with chest pain suggestive of acute myocardial infarction (AMI) and:

- ST segment elevation > 0·2 mV in 2 adjacent chest leads, or > 0·1 mV in 2 or more 'adjacent' limb leads; **or**

- dominant R waves and ST depression in V1-V3 (posterior infarction); **or**

- new-onset (or presumed new-onset) left bundle branch block.

### Dose

The drugs and doses used for thrombolysis are discussed in Chapter 3.

### Actions and use

Thrombolytic therapy may restore the patency of an infarct-related artery and reduce left ventricular damage and remodelling. Its clinical benefit depends largely on how quickly and completely reperfusion is achieved. Thus, initiating thrombolytic therapy is almost as urgent as the treatment of cardiac arrest. It is critical to avoid any delay in thrombolytic therapy in patients with STEMI. In many health systems thrombolytic therapy is given in the emergency department. Consider prehospital thrombolytic therapy if there is delay in the transfer of patients to hospital. The choice of thrombolytic drug will depend on local protocols. Thrombolytic therapy in acute coronary syndromes is discussed in depth in Chapter 3.

## Key learning points

- The role of drugs during cardiac arrest is secondary to attempted defibrillation, effective chest compressions and effective ventilation with a high concentration of oxygen.

- There are no data to prove that any drugs used during cardiac arrest alter long-term outcome.

- Guidance on the selection of antiarrhythmic drugs is given in the peri-arrest algorithms (Chapter 12).

## Further reading

International Liaison Committee on Resuscitation. 2005 International Consensus on Cardiopulmonary Resuscitation and Emergency Cardiovascular Care Science with Treatment Recommendations. Part 4. Advanced life support. Resuscitation 2005;67:213-47.

Nolan JP, Deakin CD, Soar J, Bottiger BW, Smith G. European Resuscitation Council Guidelines for Resuscitation 2005. Section 4: Adult advanced life support. Resuscitation 2005;67 Suppl 1:S39-86.

International Liaison Committee on Resuscitation. 2005 International Consensus on Cardiopulmonary Resuscitation and Emergency Cardiovascular Care Science with Treatment Recommendations. Part 5. Acute coronary syndromes. Resuscitation 2005;67:249-69.

Arntz H-R, Bossaert L, Filippatos GS. European Resuscitation Council Guidelines for Resuscitation 2005. Section 5: Initial management of acute coronary syndromes. Resuscitation 2005;67 Suppl 1:S87-96.

ALS

# Cardiac Pacing

## CHAPTER 11

## Objectives

To understand:

▶ **The indications for cardiac pacing in the peri-arrest setting.**

▶ **How to perform percussion (fist) pacing.**

▶ **How to apply non-invasive, transcutaneous electrical pacing.**

▶ **The problems associated with temporary transvenous pacing and how to correct them.**

▶ **How to manage patients with implanted permanent pacemakers and cardioverter defibrillators in the setting of cardiac arrest and in the peri-arrest setting.**

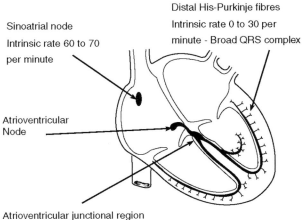

Figure 11.1 The cardiac conducting system and rates of spontaneous depolarisation

## Introduction

In some cardiac arrest or peri-arrest settings, non-invasive pacing maintains cardiac output temporarily whilst expert help is obtained to deliver longer-term treatment. Non-invasive pacing can be established rapidly and is well within the capabilities of an ALS provider.

The ALS provider does not need to have a detailed technical knowledge of permanent cardiac pacemakers and implanted cardioverter defibrillators but needs to be able to recognise when either of these devices is failing and how the presence of an implanted device may influence the management of a cardiac arrest.

## The cardiac impulse - its formation and its failure

The electrical activity that stimulates each normal heartbeat arises in the sino-atrial (SA) node. This depolarises spontaneously and regularly without any external stimulus. Such behaviour is termed automaticity, and any cardiac tissue that possesses it is capable of initiating a heartbeat and behaving as the heart's natural pacemaker. Different parts of the conducting system depolarise spontaneously at different rates (Figure 11.1). The fastest pacemaker will provide the cardiac rhythm and slower natural pacemakers will only take over if the faster ones fail. Examples may be seen in sinus arrest or extreme sinus bradycardia when the atrioventricular (AV) node may take over and provide a junctional escape rhythm, and in complete atrioventricular block (complete heart block - CHB) when the escape rhythm arises from the ventricular myocardium or from conducting tissue below the atrioventricular node.

When CHB occurs at the level of the AV node, the most rapid automatic activity arises from cells immediately below the block and these become the new pacemaker. The intrinsic rate of these cells is relatively fast (often about 50 beats min⁻¹). The resulting escape rhythm is usually relatively stable and unlikely to fail and cause asystole.

The QRS complexes resulting from this type of block are narrow since the impulse is transmitted to the ventricles rapidly through an intact His-Purkinje system. This situation may be seen complicating acute inferior myocardial infarction, where the blood supply to the AV node is impaired. In this setting narrow-complex CHB may not require pacing, as the heart rate is often not especially slow, and the risk of asystole is usually low.

Complete heart block can occur lower in the conducting system, for example when all the fibres of the bundle branches are involved following anteroseptal myocardial infarction, or as a result of other disease including degenerative fibrosis and valve disease. Any automatic activity arising below this block in the distal Purkinje fibres is likely to be slow and unreliable. In this situation, the resulting QRS complexes will be broad, since the impulse passes slowly through ventricular muscle rather then rapidly through the His-Purkinje system. The unreliable escape rhythm may fail briefly, leading to syncope (Stokes-Adams attack), or completely, causing ventricular standstill and cardiac arrest. Broad-complex CHB requires cardiac pacing, and the occurrence of significant ventricular pauses makes this urgent, as this implies a risk of asystole. The possible risk of more severe AV block and asystole should always be considered in a patient who has presented with syncope and has any ECG evidence of conduction delay (e.g., long PR interval or bundle branch block). Such patients require at least cardiac monitoring and expert assessment.

In the peri-arrest setting, artificial pacemakers are used when the cardiac rhythm is unduly slow or unreliable and not responding to the treatment described in the peri-arrest algorithm for bradycardia (Chapter 12). However, pacing will be successful only if the heart is able to respond to the pacing stimulus. In the setting of cardiac arrest the continued presence of P waves makes this more likely.

Pacing is very rarely successful in asystole in the absence of P waves and should not be attempted routinely in this situation.

The stimulus to the myocardium may be either mechanical, as in percussion pacing, or electrical as in transcutaneous and transvenous pacing.

If a pacing stimulus induces an immediate QRS complex this is referred to as 'capture'. Always check that electrical activity seen on the ECG is accompanied by mechanical activity producing a palpable pulse.

# Methods of pacing

Methods of pacing are classified as:

**Non-invasive**

- Percussion pacing ('fist pacing')

- Transcutaneous pacing

**Invasive**

- Temporary transvenous pacing

- Permanent pacing with an implanted pacemaker

Implanted devices that deliver pacing include pacemakers implanted for the treatment of bradycardia, biventricular pacemakers implanted for the treatment of heart failure (cardiac resynchronisation therapy) and implanted cardioverter defibrillators that also have a pacemaker function.

## Non-invasive Pacing

### Percussion pacing

When bradycardia is so profound that it causes clinical cardiac arrest, percussion pacing can be used in preference to CPR since it is capable of producing an adequate cardiac output with minimal trauma to the patient. It is most likely to be successful when ventricular standstill is accompanied by continuing P wave activity (Chapter 7).

### How to perform percussion pacing

- Deliver repeated firm but gentle blows over the precordium lateral to the lower left sternal edge.

- Raise the hand only about 10 cm above the chest for each blow.

- These blows should be just gentle enough to be tolerated by a conscious patient.

- If initial blows do not produce a QRS complex try to find the best position for percussion by moving the point of contact around the precordium until a site is found that produces repeated ventricular stimulation.

- If necessary, reduce the force of the blows until a threshold is found below which a blow is too gentle to stimulate a QRS complex.

Percussion pacing is not as reliable as electrical pacing in stimulating QRS complexes. If percussion does not produce a pulsed rhythm promptly, regardless of whether or not it stimulates QRS complexes, start CPR without further delay.

Like CPR, percussion pacing is an emergency measure that is used to try to maintain circulation to vital organs and enable either recovery of a spontaneous cardiac rhythm or transcutaneous or transvenous pacing.

### Transcutaneous pacing

Compared to transvenous pacing, non-invasive transcutaneous pacing has the following advantages:

- it can be established very quickly;

- it is easy to perform and requires a minimum of training;

- it avoids the risks of central venous cannulation;

- it can be initiated by nurses, paramedics and doctors, while waiting for expert help to establish transvenous pacing.

The major disadvantage of transcutaneous pacing in the conscious patient is discomfort. The pacing impulse stimulates painful contraction of chest wall muscles as well as causing some direct discomfort. Many defibrillators incorporate a facility for transcutaneous pacing but stand-alone non-invasive pacing devices are also available. The development of multifunction, adhesive electrode pads capable of ECG monitoring, pacing, cardioversion, and defibrillation have made these units particularly easy to use.

Most modern transcutaneous pacing systems are capable of demand pacing: intrinsic QRS complexes are sensed and pacing stimuli delivered only when needed.

### How to perform transcutaneous pacing

- Despite the need to start pacing without delay, careful attention to technique will increase the chance of success.

- Using scissors or a razor, quickly remove excess chest hair from the skin where the electrode pad is to be applied.

- Make sure that the skin is dry.

- Attach ECG monitoring electrodes and leads if necessary - these are needed with some transcutaneous pacing devices.

- Position the electrode pads in the anterior-posterior (A-P) positions if possible (Figures 11.2a-c). This is usually possible in a 'peri-arrest' setting.

- If the pacing device is not capable of defibrillation, defibrillator pads or paddles can still be used in the 'conventional' right pectoral and apical positions if cardiac arrest occurs.

- If the pacing device is part of a defibrillator, a defibrillatory shock can be delivered effectively using A-P positions should it be required.

- If applying pads during cardiac arrest use right pectoral and apical positions (Figure 11.2d): chest compressions should not be interrupted to allow placement of a posterior electrode.

- Check that the polarity of pacing electrodes and cables is correct and complies with the manufacturer's instructions: if the polarity is reversed, failure to capture or high pacing thresholds may result.

- For A-P positions place the anterior electrode on the left anterior chest wall, beside the sternum, overlying the V2 and V3 ECG electrode positions. Place the posterior electrode between the lower part of the left scapula and the spine, at the same horizontal level on the trunk as the anterior electrode.

- The electrodes of multifunction pacing-defibrillator devices can also be placed in the anterior-posterior positions, but during cardiac arrest it is more convenient to use the right pectoral-apical configuration (Figure 11.2d) as chest compressions do not have to be interrupted to turn the patient to place the posterior electrode. Place one electrode to the right of the upper sternum below the clavicle. The apical pad is placed in the mid-axillary line, approximately level with the V6 ECG electrode or female breast. This position should be clear of any breast tissue. It is important that this electrode is placed sufficiently laterally.

- Select demand mode if available and adjust the ECG gain to enable sensing of any intrinsic QRS complexes. If there is a lot of movement artefact on the ECG this may inhibit the pacemaker. Avoid movement artefact as far as possible. Otherwise a fixed-rate pacing mode will be needed.

- Select an appropriate pacing rate. This will usually be in the range of 60-90 min⁻¹ for adults, but in some circumstances (for example complete AV block with an idioventricular rhythm at 50 min⁻¹) a slower pacing rate of 40 or even 30 min⁻¹ may be appropriate to deal with sudden ventricular standstill or more extreme bradycardia.

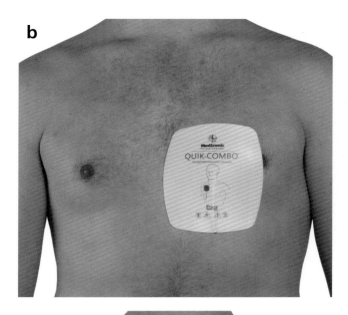

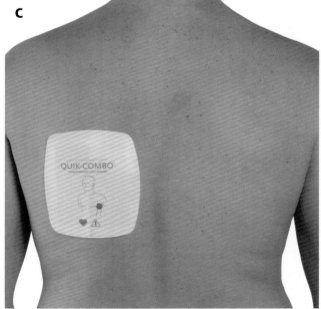

**a**

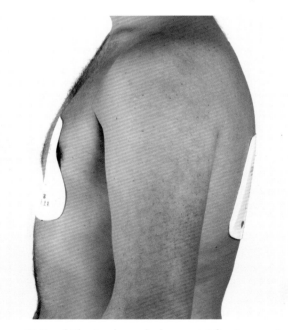

**d**

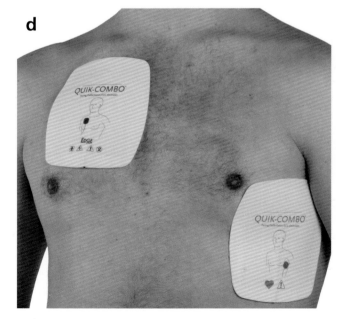

**Figures 11.2 a-d Electrode pad placement for transcutaneous pacing**

- Set the pacing current at its lowest setting and turn on the pacemaker. Gradually increase the current while observing the patient and the ECG. As the current is increased the muscles of the chest wall will contract with each impulse and a pacing spike will appear on the ECG (Figure 11.3a). Increase the current until each pacing spike is followed immediately by a QRS complex, indicating electrical capture (typically with a current of 50-100 mA). This means that the pacing stimuli are causing depolarisation of the ventricles (Figure 11.3b).

- Check that the apparent QRS complex is followed by a T wave. Occasionally, artefact generated by the pacing current travelling through the chest may be mistaken for a QRS complex, but such artefact will not be followed by a T wave (Figure 11.3a).

- If the highest current setting is reached and electrical capture has not occurred, try changing the electrode positions. Continued failure to achieve electrical capture suggests a non-viable myocardium.

Having achieved electrical capture with the pacemaker, check for a pulse. A palpable pulse confirms the presence of 'mechanical capture' (i.e., contraction of the myocardium). Failure to achieve mechanical capture in the presence of good electrical capture constitutes pulseless electrical activity (PEA). The most likely cause is severe myocardial failure but consider other possible causes of PEA in these circumstances.

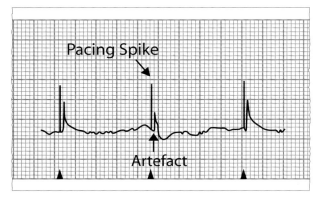
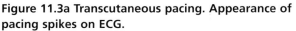

**Figure 11.3a Transcutaneous pacing. Appearance of pacing spikes on ECG.**

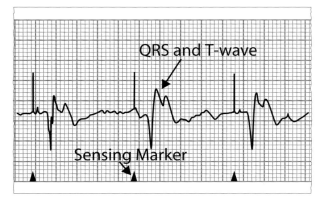

**Figure 11.3b Transcutaneous pacing. ECG shows ventricular capture after each pacing spike.**

Conscious patients usually experience considerable discomfort during transcutaneous pacing. Warn patients in advance that this may happen. They will often require intravenous analgesia and/or sedation if prolonged transcutaneous pacing is necessary.

When defibrillating a patient who has pacing-only electrode pads in place, apply the defibrillator paddles at least 2-3 cm from the pacing electrodes to prevent arcing of the defibrillation current.

Chest compressions can be given with transcutaneous electrodes in place. There is no hazard to the person doing chest compressions (less than one joule is delivered and the electrode pads are well insulated). However, there is no benefit in maintaining attempted pacing during chest compressions, so it is best to turn off the pacemaker.

When transcutaneous pacing produces an adequate cardiac output seek expert help immediately to insert a temporary transvenous pacing lead.

## Invasive pacing

### Temporary transvenous pacing

It is rare to have to attempt to insert a transvenous pacing wire during a cardiac arrest. In this setting, use non-invasive pacing to attempt to establish a cardiac output, and then seek expert help for transvenous pacing.

Failure of an existing temporary transvenous pacing system may cause cardiac arrest, particularly when the patient is pacing-dependent. Temporary transvenous pacing systems can fail in three ways:

### 1. High threshold

When a temporary pacing lead is inserted the aim is to position its tip in the apex of the right ventricle, where it is least likely to be displaced. After positioning the lead, it is used to pace the heart and the voltage delivered by the pacemaker is decreased and increased to establish the minimum voltage needed to stimulate the ventricle. This is termed the pacing threshold and the usual aim is to achieve a threshold of less than 1 V at the time of lead insertion. Higher thresholds suggest that the electrode is not making satisfactory contact with the myocardium, and the lead may need to be repositioned.

It is usual to pace the heart with a 3-4 V stimulus, well above the usual initial pacing threshold. Over the first month after insertion of a pacing lead (temporary or permanent) a rise in the threshold can be expected.

Check the threshold on temporary pacing leads at least daily to make sure that the output of the pacemaker is well above the threshold. If not, loss of capture may occur. This

ALS

is seen on the ECG as a pacing spike without a subsequent QRS complex. Loss of capture may be intermittent, so any apparent 'missed beat' of this nature should prompt a repeat check of the pacing threshold.

If loss of capture occurs because of a high threshold, immediately increase the output of the pacemaker to well above the threshold. A sudden increase in pacing threshold may be caused by lead displacement, so obtain prompt expert help, as repositioning of the lead may be required.

In some hospitals, doctors who are not experienced in the placement of endocardial pacing leads may use other types of transvenous pacing lead in an emergency. Specifically, a pacing lead attached to a flotation catheter may be used to achieve cardiac pacing, sometimes without the use of radiographic screening. As these leads do not necessarily make good, direct contact with the endocardium, the pacing threshold is usually substantially higher than with an endocardial lead.

### 2. Loss of electrical continuity

Modern temporary transvenous pacing leads are bipolar. One electrode is at the tip of the lead and the second is about 1 cm proximal to the tip. Each electrode is connected by the lead to separate connectors at the other end, outside the patient. These are usually inserted into sockets at one end of a connecting cable that in turn is connected to the terminals of the pacemaker.

Make sure that all connections between the lead and the pacemaker are making good secure contact that is unlikely to be lost easily, for example by minor movement of the lead or cable.

Loss of contact at any point will stop delivery of the pacing stimulus to the heart, seen on the ECG as absence of a pacing spike. This may be intermittent and symptomless, or may be sudden and total and may cause syncope or cardiac arrest in ventricular standstill. When pacing failure is accompanied by loss of the pacing spike on the ECG, check all connections immediately; check that the pacemaker has not been turned off inadvertently and check that its batteries are not depleted. If no such cause is present another possible explanation is a fracture of a wire within its insulation. This usually causes intermittent pacing failure and the fracture is more likely to be in the connecting cable than in the pacing lead. If this is suspected change the connecting cable immediately.

### 3. Electrode displacement

The tip of an endocardial transvenous pacing lead is usually positioned in the apex of the right ventricle. There should be enough slack in the lead as it passes through the right atrium to allow for changes in posture and deep inspiration, but not so much as to encourage displacement of the lead tip.

The tip of a pacing lead may also perforate the wall of the right ventricle and enter the pericardium with little or no apparent change in position on chest X-ray. Rarely, this may cause pericardial tamponade, so consider this possibility if a patient with a recently implanted pacing lead suffers cardiac arrest with pulseless electrical activity.

When displacement or perforation occurs, the ECG will still show a pacing spike, but there is likely to be intermittent or complete loss of capture of the pacing stimulus, so the pacing spikes are not followed consistently by QRS complexes. When a pacing lead displaces but remains in the right ventricle it may trigger ventricular extrasystoles or more serious ventricular arrhythmia, including VT and VF. When transvenous pacing fails, there is a risk of cardiac arrest in ventricular standstill. This may be relatively short-lived and cause syncope, or prolonged and cause cardiac arrest. In this situation use non-invasive pacing until effective transvenous pacing has been re-established.

## Implanted permanent pacing systems

Problems with permanent pacing systems are rare, because the connections between pacing electrodes and the pacemaker are much more secure. Occasional fracture of a permanent pacing lead may occur, usually following trauma such as a fall on to an outstretched arm on the side of the pacemaker. This may cause permanent or intermittent loss of the pacing spike.

If a patient with an implanted permanent pacemaker suffers cardiac arrest or requires cardioversion, place defibrillator paddles or self-adhesive pads at least 12-15 cm from the pacemaker. Pacemakers are often implanted below the left clavicle and present no problem with the use of standard defibrillator paddle positions. If a pacemaker has been implanted below the right clavicle, use A-P positions for defibrillation or cardioversion if possible. This is most easily and safely achieved using hands-free adhesive electrode pads rather than hand-held defibrillator paddles.

Automated external defibrillators (AEDs) may interpret the pacing spike of a pacemaker incorrectly as an ECG complex and consequently fail to detect a shockable rhythm.

## Biventricular pacing systems

Until relatively recently, the usual reason for implantation of a permanent pacemaker has been the treatment of bradycardia, caused mostly by malfunction of the sino-atrial node or atrioventricular conduction. Recently, there has been increasing use of biventricular pacemakers as 'cardiac resynchronisation therapy' in patients with heart failure. Most of these patients do not require pacing for bradycardia. Pacing the apex of the right ventricle and the lateral wall of the left ventricle simultaneously improves the co-ordination of left ventricular contraction. These pacemakers require the same precautions during defibrillation and cardioversion as any other pacemaker, but failure of a pacemaker that has been inserted for this purpose will not usually cause any major change in heart rate or any dangerous rhythm abnormality.

ALS

# Implantable cardioverter-defibrillators (ICDs)

These devices resemble large implanted pacemakers. Many of them can function as demand pacemakers in the event of bradycardia and some will also deliver biventricular pacing for heart failure, as well as delivering defibrillation if required. National and international guidelines define indications for the implantation of an ICD, but accumulating evidence for improved survival after major myocardial infarction and in patients with heart failure will increase the use of these devices. Unlike a simple pacemaker, the primary function of an ICD is to terminate a life-threatening tachyarrhythmia. A simple ICD can deliver a defibrillatory shock when it detects VF or very fast VT. More sophisticated devices can be programmed also to deliver critically timed pacing stimuli to attempt to terminate VT that is not especially fast and is unlikely to cause cardiac arrest, resorting to defibrillation only if the VT accelerates or degenerates into VF.

ICDs are implanted usually in the pectoral region in a similar position to pacemakers. Though these devices may seem complex, the means by which they sense changes in cardiac rhythm is relatively simple, depending mainly upon detection of rapid heart rates. Consequently, ICDs will occasionally misdiagnose an arrhythmia, or misinterpret other electrical signals, and deliver inappropriate shocks, which are very unpleasant for a conscious patient. Implantable cardioverter defibrillators can be disabled temporarily by holding or taping a magnet on the skin over the device. Seek expert help if ICD malfunction is suspected, as it may require reprogramming.

If a patient who has an ICD suffers a cardiac arrest that is not terminated by the ICD, deliver CPR in the usual way. This can be performed without risk to the rescuer, even if the ICD delivers an internal shock to the patient during chest compression. If a shockable cardiac arrest rhythm is present and is not terminated by the ICD, use external defibrillation in standard fashion, taking the same precautions with choice of defibrillator paddle positions as in a patient with an implanted pacemaker.

Consider the possible requirement for ICD implantation in any patient who has been resuscitated from cardiac arrest in a shockable rhythm outside the context of proven acute ST segment elevation myocardial infarction. All such patients should be referred before discharge from hospital for assessment by a cardiologist with expertise in heart rhythm disorders.

# Key learning points

- Non-invasive pacing is achieved easily and is the immediate treatment for bradyarrhythmia that is a potential risk to the patient and does not respond to initial drug treatment (atropine).

- Non-invasive pacing is a temporary measure to be used until either a stable and effective spontaneous rhythm returns, or a competent person establishes transvenous pacing.

- Special precautions are necessary during resuscitation attempts in patients with implanted pacemakers and ICDs.

- The possible need for an ICD should be considered in patients resuscitated from cardiac arrest in VT or VF, in whom there is a possible risk of recurrence.

# Further reading

International Liaison Committee on Resuscitation. 2005 International Consensus on Cardiopulmonary Resuscitation and Emergency Cardiovascular Care Science with Treatment Recommendations. Part 4. Advanced life support. Resuscitation 2005;67:213-47.

Deakin CD, Nolan JP. European Resuscitation Council Guidelines for Resuscitation 2005. Section 3: Electrical therapies: automated external defibrillators, defibrillation, cardioversion and pacing. Resuscitation 2005;67 Suppl 1:S25-37.

DiMarco JP. Implantable cardioverter-defibrillators. N Engl J Med 2003;349:1836-47.

ALS

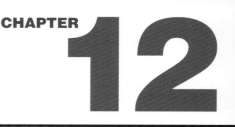
# Peri-arrest Arrhythmias

### Objectives

To understand:

▶ **The importance of arrhythmias that may precede or follow a cardiac arrest.**

▶ **How to assess peri-arrest arrhythmias.**

▶ **The principles of treatment of peri-arrest arrhythmias.**

## Introduction

The rhythm abnormalities that cause cardiac arrest require immediate treatment if resuscitation is to be successful. The recognition and treatment of these arrhythmias has been described in earlier chapters. Rhythm abnormalities can also occur after initial resuscitation from cardiac arrest and restoration of spontaneous circulation (ROSC). Rhythm abnormalities can occur in other situations without causing cardiac arrest: they are a relatively common complication of acute myocardial infarction (AMI) but are also common in patients with other cardiac abnormalities and in people who do not have coronary disease or structural heart disease.

Untreated, some of these arrhythmias may lead to cardiac arrest or to avoidable deterioration in the patient's condition. Others may require no immediate treatment.

You need to be able to recognise common arrhythmias, to be able to assess whether they require immediate treatment and to know what treatment is appropriate. This chapter focuses on common arrhythmias that may occur in the peri-arrest setting and provides guidance to enable the non-specialist ALS provider to respond safely and effectively to these in an emergency. There is a strong emphasis on the need to seek expert help with the use of more skilled or specialised treatments or when initial treatment measures are unsuccessful. If the patient is not acutely ill there is usually time to seek expert help with choosing the most appropriate treatment.

## Assessing the problem

When an arrhythmia is present or suspected, ask two basic questions:

1. How is the patient?

2. What is the rhythm?

## Assessing the patient – adverse features

For most patients the presence or absence of certain adverse symptoms or signs will dictate whether treatment is needed and the urgency to achieve control of the rhythm.

These adverse features are:

- **Clinical evidence of low cardiac output**
  Pallor, sweating, cold extremities, hypotension, drowsiness or confusion.

- **Excessive tachycardia**
  When heart rate increases diastole is shortened to a greater degree than systole. Rhythm abnormalities that cause very fast heart rates (typically > 150 min⁻¹) reduce cardiac output dramatically (because diastole is very short and the heart does not have time to fill properly) and reduce coronary blood flow (because this mostly occurs during diastole), potentially causing myocardial ischaemia. The faster the heart rate, the less well it will be tolerated.

  Broad complex tachycardias are tolerated less well than narrow complex tachycardias at the same rate, largely because broad complex tachycardia is often (but not always) associated with more severe heart disease.

- **Excessive bradycardia**
  This adverse sign is defined as a heart rate of less than 40 min⁻¹. Lesser degrees of bradycardia may be tolerated poorly by patients with severe heart disease, who cannot increase their stroke volume to compensate for the bradycardia. Some patients with very severe heart disease require faster than normal heart rates to maintain cardiac output, and even a 'normal' heart rate may be inappropriately slow for these patients.

- **Heart failure**
  Arrhythmias reduce the efficiency of the heart as a pump and may reduce coronary blood flow. Arrhythmias are a common complication of heart failure, and when they occur may precipitate heart failure or make existing heart failure worse. Left heart failure causes pulmonary oedema (breathlessness, pulmonary crackles, pulmonary oedema on chest X-ray). Right heart failure and congestive heart failure cause peripheral oedema (elevated jugular venous pressure, leg oedema, sacral oedema, hepatic congestion and enlargement).

- **Chest pain**
  The presence of chest pain implies that the arrhythmia (particularly a tachyarrhythmia) is causing myocardial ischaemia. This is especially important if there is underlying coronary artery disease or structural heart disease in which myocardial ischaemia is likely to lead to further life-threatening complications including cardiac arrest.

## Assessing the rhythm

Clinical assessment is of limited value in identifying what the rhythm abnormality is. It is usually possible to assess whether the pulse is regular or irregular and whether the heart rate is slow, normal or fast, but confident identification of cardiac rhythm is rarely possible from clinical signs alone, even by experts.

Establish rhythm monitoring as early as possible during the assessment and treatment of any arrhythmia. It is not always possible to identify cardiac rhythm accurately from a single-channel ECG monitor or recording. Whenever possible record a 12-lead ECG during the arrhythmia. This will help to identify the arrhythmia before treatment and will be available as a permanent record to guide subsequent management.

Remember always to record a 12-lead ECG **after** successful treatment of an arrhythmia as this may show abnormalities (or absence of abnormalities) that will be important in planning future management.

## Treatment

Whenever adverse features are present, give oxygen and obtain intravenous access whilst assessing the rhythm.

Having assessed the patient and the rhythm, consider other factors that may have contributed to the development of arrhythmia or may interfere with its treatment. For example, check electrolytes and correct any abnormality of potassium, magnesium or calcium concentrations.

There are then several treatment options to consider:

1.  no immediate treatment required;

2.  physical manoeuvres (e.g., vagal stimulation);

3.  anti-arrhythmic (and other) drugs;

4.  electrical cardioversion;

5.  cardiac pacing.

All anti-arrhythmic treatments (physical manoeuvres, drugs, cardioversion, pacing) have the potential to make the rhythm worse rather than better, causing clinical deterioration. Furthermore most anti-arrhythmic drugs cause myocardial depression, which may worsen heart failure or hypotension.

It is therefore important to recognise those patients who are stable and have no adverse signs from an arrhythmia. If there is no immediate urgency for treatment, and especially if there is any uncertainty about the best choice of treatment, seek expert help.

Anti-arrhythmic drugs are generally slower and less reliable than electrical cardioversion in converting a tachyarrhythmia to sinus rhythm. In general, drugs are therefore used as first-line treatment for more stable patients without adverse features and electrical cardioversion is usually the safest and most effective option for the unstable patient with adverse features.

## Electrical cardioversion

This is a relatively reliable method of terminating a tachyarrhythmia and restoring sinus rhythm in most cases. When electrical cardioversion is used to attempt to terminate a narrow-complex or broad-complex tachycardia the shock must be synchronised with the R wave of the ECG - delivery of the shock at the time of the T wave could precipitate VF. Defibrillators used for cardioversion have a switch to activate this synchronisation with the R wave.

The shock used for cardioversion is unpleasant and this treatment should always be carried out under sedation or general anaesthesia, given by an appropriately experienced doctor.

Having identified the need for cardioversion:

*   Obtain expert help immediately.

*   Ensure that IV access is adequate.

*   Attach the patient to the defibrillator – monitor through leads not pads.

*   Ensure a good quality ECG signal – change lead if necessary.

*   Press the synchronisation switch and confirm that the defibrillator is identifying the R wave correctly.

*   When the patient is sedated or anaesthetised, charge the defibrillator.

*   For choice of energy levels see below.

*   **Use all safety measures as for defibrillation** – stand clear etc.

*   Press the shock button and keep it pressed until the shock is delivered – there may be a slight delay before the shock is delivered.

*   If a second shock is needed, reactivate the synchronisation switch if necessary.

The best energy levels for defibrillation are a matter of debate and may vary according to circumstances, including the rhythm and the size of the patient. Use a biphasic defibrillator if available, as this is more likely than monophasic to achieve cardioversion with the first shock.

*   For broad complex tachycardia and AF start with 120-150 J biphasic or 200 J monophasic. If the first shock does not terminate the arrhythmia, give up to two more shocks of increasing energy up to the maximum setting of the defibrillator.

*   For atrial flutter and regular narrow complex tachycardia lower energies are usually effective. Start with 70-120 J biphasic or 100 J monophasic. If the first shock does not terminate the arrhythmia, give up to two more shocks of increasing energy up to the maximum setting of the defibrillator.

# Bradycardia

The conventional definition of bradycardia is a heart rate < 60 min$^{-1}$; however, for some people or some situations heart rates of < 60 min$^{-1}$ are not harmful and may be entirely physiological.

It is therefore helpful to distinguish:

- extreme bradycardia (< 40 min$^{-1}$)
    - rarely physiological, rarely well tolerated, and usually needs treatment
    - considered an adverse feature

- less severe bradycardia (40-60 min$^{-1}$)
    - usually needs immediate treatment only if adverse features are present

Look for adverse features and record a 12-lead ECG. The following adverse features suggest a need for immediate treatment (Figure 12.1):

- systolic BP < 90 mmHg;

- heart rate < 40 min$^{-1}$;

- ventricular arrhythmia;

- heart failure.

If any of these is present, give atropine 500 mcg intravenously. If necessary, repeat this every 3-5 min up to a total dose of 3 mg. Use atropine cautiously in the presence of acute myocardial ischaemia or acute myocardial infarction (AMI), in which atropine-induced tachycardia may worsen myocardial ischaemia or increase the size of an infarct.

If a satisfactory improvement is achieved with atropine, or if there were no adverse features requiring immediate atropine, next determine the potential risk of asystole, indicated by:

- recent asystole;

- Mobitz II atrioventricular (AV) block;

- complete AV block (3$^{rd}$ degree heart block) (especially with broad QRS or initial heart rate < 40 min$^{-1}$);

- ventricular standstill of > 3 sec.

The degrees of AV block and their significance have been described in Chapter 6.

If there is a risk of asystole, seek expert help with cardiac pacing. The definitive treatment is transvenous pacing. If there is delay in achieving this or obtaining expert help consider the temporary use of transcutaneous pacing. If this is not available or ineffective in preventing dangerous bradycardia, give adrenaline as an intravenous infusion (2-10 mcg min$^{-1}$ titrated to response).

'Fist pacing' may be used as a temporary measure to treat ventricular standstill or very extreme bradycardia whilst other treatment is being organised.

Other drugs that can be given for the treatment of bradycardia include dopamine and isoprenaline as intravenous infusions. Consider giving intravenous glucagon if a beta-blocker or calcium channel blocker is the potential cause of the bradycardia. Do not give atropine to patients with cardiac transplants as the hearts are denervated and will not respond to vagal blockade, and there is some risk of inducing paradoxical atrioventricular block.

Complete AV block with narrow QRS complexes is not an absolute indication for immediate cardiac pacing in every case - the rhythm is arising from the AV junction and may provide an adequate heart rate with a low risk of asystole, and a satisfactory response to atropine if required. The need for pacing in the longer term in these patients will depend on the underlying cause of the AV block and on whether or not it persists; for example, narrow-complex complete AV block after inferior AMI is almost always transient and very rarely needs permanent cardiac pacing. Congenital complete AV block is usually narrow-complexed and permanent pacing is usually recommended in adults to protect against a small, but definite, risk of sudden death that increases with age.

See Chapter 11 for further information about cardiac pacing, including 'fist pacing' and transcutaneous pacing.

# Tachycardia

The first step in the management of a tachyarrhythmia is the assessment of the patient (Figure 12.2).

When the pulse is absent during a tachycardia this is cardiac arrest and is NOT a peri-arrest arrhythmia. Follow the cardiac arrest algorithm to treat the patient. An exception to this rule occurs if there is a very rapid (> 250 beats min$^{-1}$) narrow-complex tachycardia (see page 116).

If a pulse is present, assess the patient for adverse features. Adverse features with a tachyarrhythmia are:

- systolic BP < 90 mmHg;

- heart rate > 150 min$^{-1}$;

- chest pain;

- heart failure;

- drowsiness or confusion;

Whilst assessing the patient:

- give oxygen and obtain IV access if not already done (particularly if adverse features are present);

- record a 12-lead ECG if not already done (without delaying treatment).

In general, at the same heart rate, a narrow-complex tachycardia causes less cardiovascular compromise than a broad-complex tachycardia.

ALS

## Bradycardia Algorithm

(includes rates inappropriately slow for haemodynamic state)

If appropriate, give oxygen, cannulate a vein, and record a 12-lead ECG

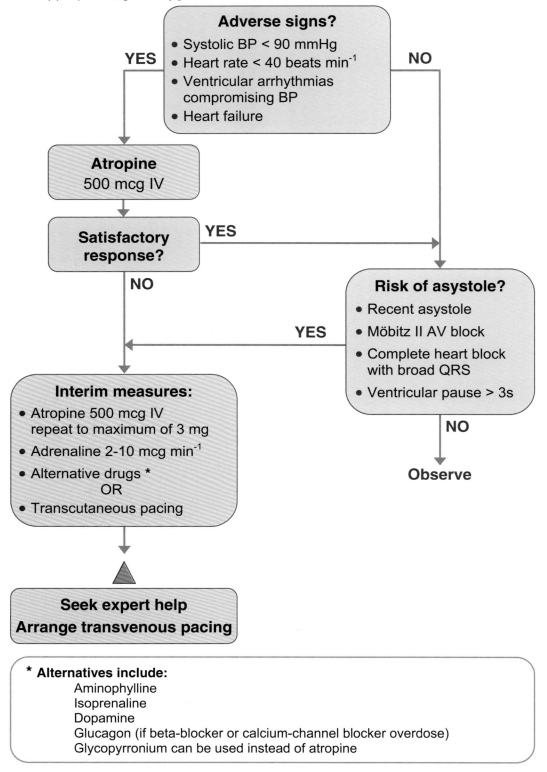

**Adverse signs?**
- Systolic BP < 90 mmHg
- Heart rate < 40 beats min$^{-1}$
- Ventricular arrhythmias compromising BP
- Heart failure

YES / NO

**Atropine**
500 mcg IV

**Satisfactory response?**

YES / NO

**Risk of asystole?**
- Recent asystole
- Möbitz II AV block
- Complete heart block with broad QRS
- Ventricular pause > 3s

YES / NO

**Observe**

**Interim measures:**
- Atropine 500 mcg IV repeat to maximum of 3 mg
- Adrenaline 2-10 mcg min$^{-1}$
- Alternative drugs *
  OR
- Transcutaneous pacing

**Seek expert help**
**Arrange transvenous pacing**

\* **Alternatives include:**
Aminophylline
Isoprenaline
Dopamine
Glucagon (if beta-blocker or calcium-channel blocker overdose)
Glycopyrronium can be used instead of atropine

**Figure 12.1 Bradycardia algorithm**

# Tachycardia Algorithm (with pulse)

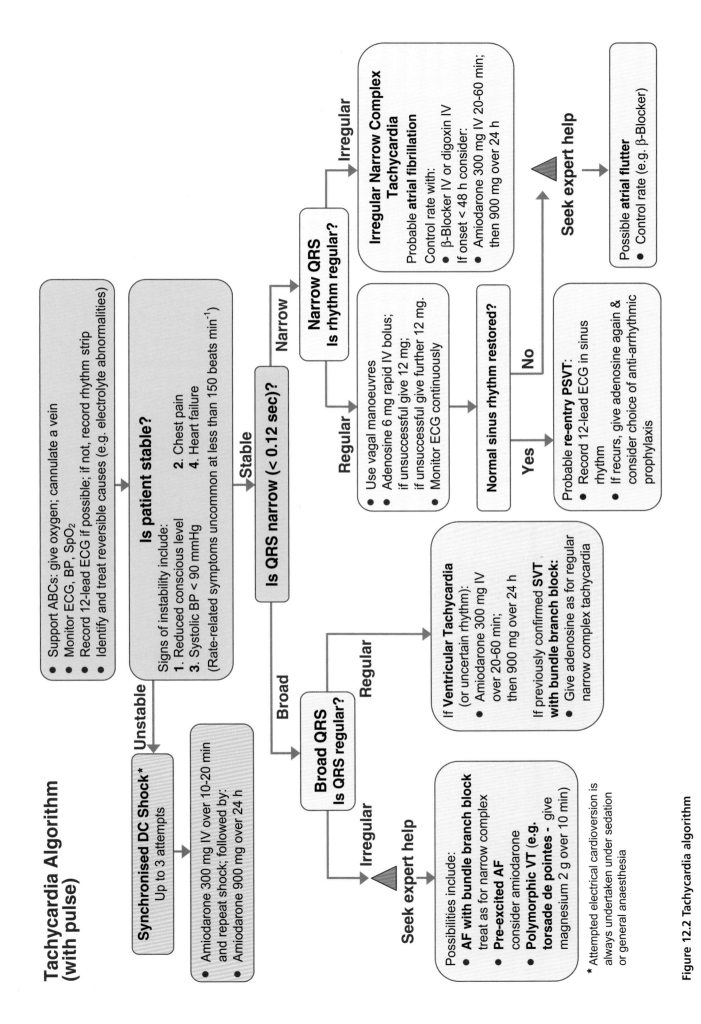

**Support ABCs: give oxygen; cannulate a vein**
- Support ABCs: give oxygen; cannulate a vein
- Monitor ECG, BP, SpO$_2$
- Record 12-lead ECG if possible; if not, record rhythm strip
- Identify and treat reversible causes (e.g. electrolyte abnormalities)

**Is patient stable?**

Signs of instability include:
1. Reduced conscious level   2. Chest pain
3. Systolic BP < 90 mmHg   4. Heart failure
(Rate-related symptoms uncommon at less than 150 beats min$^{-1}$)

**Unstable**

**Synchronised DC Shock\***
Up to 3 attempts

- Amiodarone 300 mg IV over 10-20 min and repeat shock; followed by:
- Amiodarone 900 mg over 24 h

**Stable**

**Is QRS narrow (< 0.12 sec)?**

**Broad**

**Broad QRS**
**Is QRS regular?**

**Regular**

If **Ventricular Tachycardia** (or uncertain rhythm):
- Amiodarone 300 mg IV over 20-60 min; then 900 mg over 24 h

If previously confirmed **SVT with bundle branch block**:
- Give adenosine as for regular narrow complex tachycardia

**Irregular**

**Seek expert help**

Possibilities include:
- **AF with bundle branch block** treat as for narrow complex
- **Pre-excited AF** consider amiodarone
- **Polymorphic VT (e.g. torsade de pointes** - give magnesium 2 g over 10 min)

**Narrow**

**Narrow QRS**
**Is rhythm regular?**

**Regular**

- Use vagal manoeuvres
- Adenosine 6 mg rapid IV bolus; if unsuccessful give 12 mg; if unsuccessful give further 12 mg.
- Monitor ECG continuously

**Normal sinus rhythm restored?**

**Yes**

Probable **re-entry PSVT**:
- Record 12-lead ECG in sinus rhythm
- If recurs, give adenosine again & consider choice of anti-arrhythmic prophylaxis

**No**

**Seek expert help**

Possible **atrial flutter**
- Control rate (e.g. β-Blocker)

**Irregular**

**Irregular Narrow Complex Tachycardia**

Probable **atrial fibrillation**
Control rate with:
- β-Blocker IV or digoxin IV
If onset < 48 h consider:
- Amiodarone 300 mg IV 20-60 min; then 900 mg over 24 h

\* Attempted electrical cardioversion is always undertaken under sedation or general anaesthesia

**Figure 12.2 Tachycardia algorithm**

ALS

*The following recommendations apply only to those patients in a peri-arrest situation (e.g., after initial resuscitation from cardiac arrest, following recent AMI, following the recent onset of symptomatic arrhythmia etc). They do not usually apply to patients with an established chronic arrhythmia and/or with progression of a chronic condition such as congestive heart failure (e.g., the patient with chronic atrial fibrillation and worsening chronic congestive heart failure, in whom the BP may be low, and heart failure present, but immediate cardioversion may not be appropriate).*

In the peri-arrest setting, if the patient is unstable and deteriorating with adverse features caused by the tachycardia, attempt synchronised cardioversion immediately.

If cardioversion is unsuccessful give amiodarone 300 mg intravenously over 10-20 min, then repeat attempted cardioversion. Follow the initial dose with amiodarone infusion 900 mg over 24 h.

If there are no adverse features during a tachyarrhythmia, determine whether the arrhythmia has narrow (i.e., normal duration) QRS complexes or whether they are broad (0.12 sec or longer). This distinguishes broad-complex tachycardia from narrow-complex tachycardia.

## Broad-complex tachycardia

If there are no adverse signs to indicate a need for electrical cardioversion, further assessment will help to guide the most appropriate choice of treatment.

Although broad-complex tachycardia can be a supraventricular tachycardia with aberrant conduction (i.e., bundle branch block), in the peri-arrest setting assume that broad-complex tachycardias are ventricular in origin. Treating a supraventricular tachycardia (SVT) as if it were ventricular tachycardia (VT) is less likely to lead to deterioration than treating VT as SVT. However, assessment may allow some exceptions to this approach, as detailed below.

First, examine the ECG carefully to establish whether the broad complex tachycardia is regular or irregular.

### Regular broad-complex tachycardia

In the absence of adverse features, give amiodarone 300 mg intravenously over 20-60 min, followed by an infusion of 900 mg over 24 h.

Continue to monitor and assess the patient, seek expert help, and be prepared to use electrical cardioversion if adverse features develop, or if the arrhythmia persists for several hours.

If there is clearly established evidence that the rhythm is SVT with bundle branch block, treat in the same way as regular narrow-complex tachycardia (see below). However, in case of any uncertainty, the default position is - treat as VT.

Ventricular tachycardia is more likely in the acute phase of AMI and in patients with established ischaemic heart disease.

### Irregular broad complex tachycardia

This is most likely to be atrial fibrillation (AF) with bundle branch block, but careful examination of a 12-lead ECG (if necessary by an expert) may enable confident identification of the rhythm.

Another possible cause is AF with ventricular pre-excitation, (in patients with Wolff-Parkinson-White (WPW) Syndrome)(Figure 7.9). There is more variation in the appearance and width of the QRS complexes than in AF with bundle branch block. A third possible cause is polymorphic VT (e.g., torsade de pointes (Rhythm Strip 12)), but polymorphic VT is relatively unlikely to be present without adverse features.

Seek expert help with the assessment and treatment of irregular broad-complex tachyarrhythmia. If treating AF with bundle branch block, treat as for AF (see below). If pre-excited AF (or atrial flutter) is suspected, avoid adenosine, digoxin, verapamil and diltiazem. These drugs block the AV node and cause a relative increase in pre-excitation. Electrical cardioversion is usually the safest treatment option.

Treat torsade de pointes VT immediately by stopping all drugs known to prolong the QT interval. Correct electrolyte abnormalities, especially hypokalaemia. Give magnesium sulphate 2 g intravenously over 10 min. Obtain expert help as other treatment (e.g., overdrive pacing) may be indicated to prevent relapse once the arrhythmia has been corrected. If adverse features develop (usual), arrange immediate synchronised cardioversion. If the patient becomes pulseless, attempt defibrillation immediately (cardiac arrest algorithm).

## Narrow-complex tachycardia

Regular narrow-complex tachycardias include:

- sinus tachycardia;

- AV nodal re-entry tachycardia – AVNRT (the commonest type of SVT);

- AV re-entry tachycardia - AVRT (caused by WPW Syndrome);

- atrial flutter with regular AV conduction (usually 2:1).

Irregular narrow-complex tachycardia is most commonly atrial fibrillation (AF) or sometimes atrial flutter with variable AV conduction (variable block).

### Regular narrow-complex tachycardia

#### Sinus tachycardia

This is a common physiological response to a stimulus such as exercise or anxiety. In a sick patient it may be seen in response to many stimuli such as pain, fever, anaemia, blood loss and heart failure. Treatment is almost always directed at the underlying cause — trying to slow sinus tachycardia caused by one of these conditions will make the situation worse.

## AVNRT and AVRT (paroxysmal SVT)

AV nodal re-entry tachycardia is the commonest type of paroxysmal SVT, often seen in people without any other form of heart disease and is relatively uncommon in a peri-arrest setting. It causes a regular narrow-complex tachycardia, often with no clearly visible atrial activity on the ECG, with heart rates usually well above the typical range of sinus rates at rest (60-120 min$^{-1}$). It is usually benign, unless there is additional co-incidental structural heart disease or coronary disease, but may cause symptoms that the patient finds frightening.

AV re-entry tachycardia is seen in patients with the WPW Syndrome and is also usually benign unless there happens to be additional structural heart disease. The common type of AVRT is a regular narrow-complex tachycardia, also often having no visible atrial activity on the ECG.

## Atrial flutter with regular AV conduction (often 2:1 block)

This produces a regular narrow-complex tachycardia in which it may be difficult to see atrial activity and identify flutter waves with confidence, so may be indistinguishable initially from AVNRT and AVRT.

When atrial flutter with 2:1 block or even 1:1 conduction is accompanied by bundle branch block it produces a regular broad-complex tachycardia that will usually be very difficult to distinguish from VT; treatment of this rhythm as if it were VT will usually be effective or will lead to slowing of the ventricular response and identification of the rhythm.

Most typical atrial flutter has an atrial rate of about 300 min$^{-1}$, so atrial flutter with 2:1 block tends to produce a tachycardia of about 150 min$^{-1}$ (Rhythm Strip 9). Much faster rates (170 min$^{-1}$ or more) are unlikely to be due to atrial flutter with 2:1 block.

## Treatment of regular narrow-complex tachycardia

If the patient is unstable with adverse features caused by the arrhythmia, attempt synchronised electrical cardioversion. It is reasonable to give adenosine to an unstable patient with a regular narrow-complex tachycardia, while preparations are made for synchronized cardioversion. However, do not delay electrical cardioversion if the adenosine fails to restore sinus rhythm.

In the absence of adverse features:

- Start with vagal manoeuvres. Carotid sinus massage or the Valsalva manoeuvre will terminate up to a quarter of episodes of paroxysmal SVT. A Valsalva manoeuvre

(forced expiration against a closed glottis) in the supine position may be the most effective technique. A practical way of achieving this without protracted explanation is to ask the patient to blow into a 20 ml syringe with enough force to push back the plunger. Avoid carotid massage if a carotid bruit is present; rupture of an atheromatous plaque could cause cerebral embolism and stroke. Be aware that sudden bradycardia may trigger ventricular fibrillation in the context of acute ischaemia or digitalis toxicity. Record an ECG (preferably multi-lead) during each manoeuvre. If the rhythm is atrial flutter, slowing of the ventricular response will often occur and demonstrate flutter waves.

- If the arrhythmia persists and is not atrial flutter, use adenosine. Give 6 mg as a rapid intravenous bolus. Record an ECG (preferably multi-lead) during each injection. If the ventricular rate slows transiently, but the arrhythmia then persists, look for atrial activity such as atrial flutter or other atrial tachycardia and treat accordingly. If there is no response to adenosine 6 mg give a 12 mg bolus. If there is no response give one further 12 mg bolus.

- Successful termination of a tachyarrhythmia by vagal manoeuvres or adenosine indicates that it was almost certainly AVNRT or AVRT. Monitor the patients for further rhythm abnormalities. Treat recurrence either with further adenosine or with a longer-acting drug with AV nodal blocking action (e.g., diltiazem or beta blocker).

- Vagal manoeuvres or adenosine will terminate almost all AVNRT or AVRT within seconds. Failure to terminate a regular narrow-complex tachycardia with adenosine suggests an atrial tachycardia such as atrial flutter.

- If adenosine is contra-indicated or fails to terminate a regular narrow-complex tachycardia without demonstrating that it is atrial flutter, give a calcium channel blocker (e.g., verapamil 2.5-5 mg IV over 2 min; or diltiazem 15-20 mg over 2 min).

## Irregular narrow-complex tachycardia

An irregular narrow-complex tachycardia is most likely to be AF with an uncontrolled ventricular response (Rhythm Strip 6) or less commonly atrial flutter with variable AV block. Record a 12-lead ECG to identify the rhythm (Chapter 6).

If the patient is unstable with adverse features caused by the arrhythmia, attempt synchronised electrical cardioversion.

If there are no adverse features, treatment options include:

- rate control by drug therapy;

- rhythm control using drugs to encourage chemical cardioversion;

- rhythm control by electrical cardioversion;

- treatment to prevent complications (e.g., anticoagulation).

Obtain expert help to determine the most appropriate treatment for the individual patient.

The longer a patient remains in AF the greater is the likelihood of atrial clot developing. In general, patients who have been in AF for more than 48 h should not be treated by cardioversion (electrical or chemical) until they have been fully anticoagulated or unless absence of atrial clot has been shown by trans-oesophageal echocardiography.

If the aim is to control heart rate, options include a beta-blocker, digoxin, diltiazem, magnesium, or combinations of these.

If the duration of AF is less than 48 h and rhythm control is considered appropriate, this may be attempted using amiodarone (300 mg intravenously over 20-60 min followed by 900 mg over 24 h). Ibutilide or flecainide can also be given for rhythm control, but expert advice should be obtained before using these drugs for this purpose. Electrical cardioversion remains an option in this setting and will restore sinus rhythm in more patients than chemical cardioversion.

Seek expert help if any patient with AF is known or found to have ventricular pre-excitation (WPW Syndrome). Avoid using adenosine, diltiazem, verapamil or digoxin for patients with pre-excited AF or atrial flutter as these block the AV node and cause a relative increase in pre-excitation.

### Rapid narrow-complex tachycardia with no pulse

Rarely, a very rapid (usually > 250 beats min[-1]) narrow-complex tachycardia can impair cardiac output to such an extent that the pulse may be impalpable and consciousness impaired. The appropriate treatment is immediate synchronised cardioversion.

## Key learning points

- Arrhythmias occurring after resuscitation from cardiac arrest and ROSC may need treatment to stabilise the patient and prevent recurrence of cardiac arrest.

- In other settings some arrhythmias may require prompt treatment to prevent deterioration, including risk of cardiac arrest, and others do not require immediate treatment.

- The urgency for treatment and the best choice of treatment is determined by the condition of the patient (adverse features) and by the nature of the arrhythmia.

- Obtain expert help with the assessment and treatment of cardiac arrhythmia as soon as possible.

## Further reading

Blomstrom-Lundqvist C, Scheinmann M M et al. American College of Cardiology/American Heart Association Task Force and the European Society of Cardiology Committee for Practice Guidelines. ACC/AHA/ESC Guidelines for the Management of Patients With Supraventricular Arrhythmias. European Heart Journal 2003;24:1857-97.

Fuster V, Lyden R E et al. American College of Cardiology/American Heart Association Task Force and the European Society of Cardiology Committee for Practice Guidelines and Policy Conferences. ACC/AHA/ESC guidelines for the management of patients with atrial fibrillation. European Heart Journal 2001;22:1852-1923.

# Cardiac Arrest in Special Circumstances

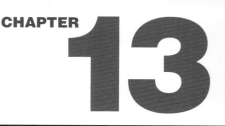

## Introduction

Resuscitation needs to be modified in specific circumstances. Early recognition of signs and symptoms and effective treatment will often prevent cardiac arrest. These conditions account for a large proportion of cardiac arrests in younger patients with no co-existing disease.

## Life-threatening electrolyte disorders

Electrolyte abnormalities can cause cardiac arrhythmias or cardiorespiratory arrest. Potassium disorders pose the greatest risk. Consider starting treatment in life-threatening electrolyte disorders before laboratory results are available. Electrolyte values for definitions are quoted as a guide to clinical decision-making. The precise values that trigger treatment decisions will depend on the patient's clinical condition and rate of change of electrolyte values.

### Prevention of electrolyte disorders

- Treat life-threatening electrolyte abnormalities before cardiac arrest occurs.

- Remove precipitating factors (e.g., drugs) and monitor electrolyte concentrations to prevent recurrence of the abnormality.

- Monitor renal function in patients at risk of electrolyte disorders.

- Review renal replacement therapy (e.g., haemodialysis) regularly to avoid inappropriate electrolyte shifts during treatment.

## Potassium disorders

### Potassium homeostasis

Extracellular potassium concentration is regulated tightly between 3.5 and 5.0 mmol $l^{-1}$. A large concentration gradient normally exists between intracellular and extracellular fluid compartments. Evaluation of serum potassium must take into consideration the effects of changes in serum pH. When serum pH decreases, serum potassium concentration increases, because potassium shifts from the cellular to the vascular space. When serum pH increases, serum potassium concentration decreases because potassium shifts into cells. Anticipate the effects of pH changes on serum potassium during therapy for hyperkalaemia or hypokalaemia.

### Hyperkalaemia

Hyperkalaemia is usually caused by increased potassium release from cells or impaired excretion by the kidneys.

#### Definition

There is no universal definition. We have defined hyperkalaemia as a serum potassium concentration higher than 5.5 mmol $l^{-1}$; in practice, hyperkalaemia is a continuum. As the potassium concentration increases, the risk of adverse events increases and the need for urgent treatment increases. Severe hyperkalaemia has been defined as a serum potassium concentration higher than 6.5 mmol $l^{-1}$.

#### Causes

The causes of hyperkalaemia include:

- renal failure;

- drugs (angiotensin converting enzyme inhibitors (ACEI), angiotensin II receptor blockers (ARB), potassium sparing diuretics, non-steroidal anti-inflammatory drugs (NSAIDs), beta-blockers, trimethoprim);

- tissue breakdown (skeletal muscle (rhabdomyolysis), tumour lysis, haemolysis);

- metabolic acidosis;

- endocrine disorders (Addison's disease);

- hyperkalaemic periodic paralysis;

- diet (may be the principal cause in patients receiving chronic renal replacement therapy).

Abnormal erythrocytes or thrombocytosis may cause a spuriously high potassium concentration. The risk of hyperkalaemia increases when there is a combination of causative factors.

## Recognition of hyperkalaemia

Exclude hyperkalaemia in patients with an arrhythmia or cardiac arrest. Patients may present with weakness progressing to flaccid paralysis, paraesthesia, or depressed deep tendon reflexes. The effect of hyperkalaemia on the ECG depends on the absolute serum potassium concentration as well as the rate of increase (Figure 13.1).

ECG changes with hyperkalaemia are usually progressive and include:

- first degree heart block (prolonged PR interval) (> 0.2 sec);

- flattened or absent P waves;

- tall, peaked (tented) T waves (T wave larger than R wave in more than one lead);

- ST-segment depression;

- S and T wave merging;

- widened QRS (> 0.12 sec);

- bradycardia (sinus bradycardia or AV block);

- ventricular tachycardia;

- cardiac arrest (asystole, VF/VT, PEA).

## Treatment of hyperkalaemia

The five key steps in treating hyperkalaemia are:

1. Cardiac protection by antagonising the effects of hyperkalaemia.

2. Shifting potassium into cells.

3. Removing potassium from the body.

4. Monitoring serum potassium concentration for rebound hyperkalaemia.

5. Prevention of recurrence of hyperkalaemia.

When hyperkalaemia is strongly suspected, e.g., in the presence of ECG changes, start life-saving treatment even before laboratory results are available.

### *Patient not in cardiac arrest*

Assess fluid status; if hypovolaemic, give fluid to enhance urinary potassium excretion. The values for classification are an approximate guide.

*Mild elevation (5.5-6 mmol l⁻¹): remove potassium from the body with*

- Potassium exchange resins - calcium resonium 15-30 g OR sodium polystyrene sulfonate (Kayexalate) 15-30 g in 50-100 ml of 20 % sorbitol, given either orally or by retention enema (onset in 1-3 h; maximal effect at 6 h), or

- Diuretics: furosemide 1 mg kg⁻¹ IV slowly (onset with the diuresis), or

- Consider dialysis: haemodialysis is more efficient than peritoneal dialysis at removing potassium (immediate onset; 25-30 mmol potassium h⁻¹ removed with haemodialysis).

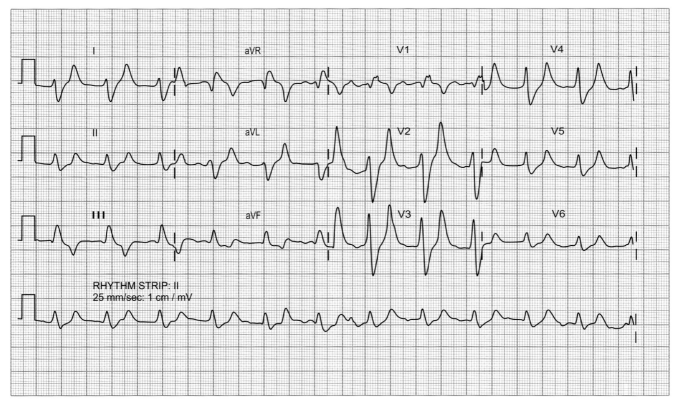

**Figure 13.1 12-lead ECG showing features of hyperkalaemia**

*Moderate elevation (6-6.5 mmol l$^{-1}$) without ECG changes: use strategies above plus shift potassium into cells with:*

- Dextrose/insulin:  10 units short-acting Insulin and 50 g glucose IV over 15-30 min (onset in 15-30 min; maximal effect at 30-60 min; monitor blood glucose).

*Severe elevation ( ≥ 6.5 mmol l$^{-1}$) without ECG changes: shift potassium into cells with strategies above plus:*

- Salbutamol: 5 mg nebulised. Several doses may be required (onset in 15-30 min).

- Sodium bicarbonate: 50 mmol IV over 5 min if metabolic acidosis present (onset in 15-30 min). Bicarbonate alone is less effective than glucose plus insulin or nebulised salbutamol; it is best used in conjunction with these medications.

*Severe elevation (≥ 6.5 mmol/l) WITH toxic ECG changes (Figure 13.1): protect the heart first with:*

- Calcium chloride: 10 ml 10% calcium chloride IV over 2-5 min to antagonise the toxic effects of hyperkalaemia at the myocardial cell membrane. This protects the heart by reducing the risk of VF, but does not lower serum potassium (onset in 1-3 min). Use in addition to potassium removal and shifting strategies stated above.

### Patient in cardiac arrest

*Modifications to BLS*

There are no modifications to basic life support in the presence of electrolyte abnormalities.

*Modifications to ALS*

Follow the universal algorithm. The general approach to treatment depends on the degree of hyperkalaemia, rate of rise of serum potassium and the patient's clinical condition.

*Cardiopulmonary arrest: protect the heart first; then use shifting and removal strategies*

- Calcium chloride: 10 ml 10% calcium chloride IV by rapid bolus injection to antagonise the toxic effects of hyperkalaemia at the myocardial cell membrane.

- Sodium bicarbonate: 50 mmol IV by rapid injection (if severe acidosis or renal failure).

- Dextrose/Insulin: 10 units short-acting insulin and 50 g glucose IV by rapid injection.

- Haemodialysis: consider this for cardiac arrest induced by hyperkalaemia which is resistant to medical treatment.

### Indications for dialysis

Haemodialysis is the most effective method of removal of potassium from the body. The typical decline in serum potassium is 1 mmol l$^{-1}$ in the first 60 min, followed by 1 mmol l$^{-1}$ over the next 2 h. Consider haemodialysis early for hyperkalaemia associated with established renal failure, oliguric acute renal failure (<400ml day$^{-1}$ urine output) or when there is marked tissue breakdown. Dialysis is also indicated when hyperkalaemia is resistant to medical management. Serum potassium concentration frequently rebounds after initial treatment.

## Hypokalaemia

Hypokalaemia is common in hospital patients. Hypokalaemia increases the incidence of arrhythmias, particularly in patients with pre-existing heart disease and in those treated with digoxin.

### Definition

Hypokalaemia is defined as serum potassium < 3.5 mmol l$^{-1}$. Severe hypokalaemia is defined as K$^+$ < 2.5 mmol l$^{-1}$ and may be associated with symptoms.

### Causes

Causes of hypokalaemia include:

- gastrointestinal loss (diarrhoea);

- drugs (diuretics, laxatives, steroids, adrenaline, isoprenaline, etc);

- renal losses (renal tubular disorders, diabetes insipidus, dialysis);

- endocrine disorders (Cushing's Syndrome, hyperaldosteronism);

- metabolic alkalosis;

- magnesium depletion;

- poor dietary intake.

Treatment for hyperkalaemia may also induce hypokalaemia.

### Recognition of hypokalaemia

Exclude hypokalaemia in every patient with an arrhythmia or cardiac arrest. In dialysis patients, hypokalaemia occurs commonly at the end of a haemodialysis session or during treatment with continuous ambulatory peritoneal dialysis (CAPD).

As serum potassium concentration decreases, the nerves and muscles are predominantly affected, causing fatigue, weakness, leg cramps, constipation. In severe cases (K$^+$< 2.5 mmol l$^{-1}$), rhabdomyolysis, ascending paralysis and respiratory difficulties may occur.

ECG features of hypokalaemia are:

- U waves;

- T wave flattening;

- ST segment changes;

- arrhythmias;

- cardiorespiratory arrest  (VF/VT, asystole, PEA).

**Treatment**

This depends on the severity of hypokalaemia and the presence of symptoms and ECG abnormalities. Gradual replacement of potassium is preferable, but in an emergency intravenous potassium is required. The maximum recommended IV infusion rate of potassium is 20 mmol h$^{-1}$, but more rapid infusion (e.g. 2 mmol min$^{-1}$ for 10 min, followed by 10 mmol over 5-10 min) is indicated for unstable arrhythmias when cardiac arrest is imminent or has occurred. Continuous ECG monitoring is essential during IV infusion. Adjust the dose after repeated sampling of serum potassium levels.

Patients who are potassium deficient can also be deficient in magnesium. Repletion of magnesium stores will facilitate more rapid correction of hypokalaemia and is recommended in severe cases of hypokalaemia.

## Calcium and magnesium disorders

The recognition and management of calcium and magnesium disorders is summarised in Table 13.1.

| DISORDER | CAUSES | PRESENTATION | ECG | TREATMENT |
|---|---|---|---|---|
| **Hypercalcaemia**<br><br><br>[Ca$^{2+}$] > 2.6 mmol l$^{-1}$ | Primary or tertiary hyperparathyroidism<br>Malignancy<br>Sarcoidosis<br>Drugs | Confusion<br>Weakness<br>Abdominal pain<br>Hypotension<br>Arrhythmias<br>Cardiac arrest | Short QT interval<br>Prolonged QRS Interval<br>Flat T waves<br>AV block<br>Cardiac arrest | Fluid replacement IV<br>Furosemide 1mg kg$^{-1}$ IV<br>Hydrocortisone 200-300 mg IV<br>Pamidronate 60-90 mg IV<br>Calcitonin 4-8 units kg$^{-1}$ 8h$^{-1}$ IM<br>Review medication<br>Haemodialysis |
| **Hypocalcaemia**<br><br><br>[Ca$^{2+}$] < 2.1 mmol l$^{-1}$ | Chronic renal failure<br>Acute pancreatitis<br>Calcium channel blocker overdose<br>Toxic shock syndrome<br>Rhabdomyolysis<br>Tumour lysis syndrome | Paraesthesia<br>Tetany<br>Seizures<br>AV- block<br>Cardiac arrest | Prolonged QT interval<br>T wave inversion<br>Heart block<br>Cardiac arrest | Calcium chloride 10% 10-40 ml IV<br>Magnesium sulphate 50% 4-8 mmol (if necessary) IV |
| **Hypermagnesaemia**<br><br><br>[Mg$^{2+}$] > 1.1 mmol l$^{-1}$ | Renal failure<br>Iatrogenic | Confusion<br>Weakness<br>Respiratory depression<br>AV-block<br>Cardiac arrest | Prolonged PR and QT intervals<br>T wave peaking<br>AV- block<br>Cardiac arrest | Calcium chloride 10% 5-10ml IV repeated if necessary<br>Ventilatory support if necessary<br>Saline diuresis – 0.9% saline with furosemide 1mg kg$^{-1}$ IV<br>Haemodialysis |
| **Hypomagnesaemia**<br><br><br>[Mg$^{2+}$] < 0.6 mmol l$^{-1}$ | GI loss<br>Polyuria<br>Starvation<br>Alcoholism<br>Malabsorption | Tremor<br>Ataxia<br>Nystagmus<br>Seizures<br>Arrhythmias – torsade de pointes<br>Cardiac arrest | Prolonged PR and QT Intervals<br>ST-segment depression<br>T-wave inversion<br>Flattened P waves<br>Increased QRS duration<br>Torsade de pointes | Severe or symptomatic:<br>2 g 50% magnesium sulphate (4 ml; 8 mmol) IV over 15 min.<br>Torsade de pointes:<br>2 g 50% magnesium sulphate (4 ml; 8 mmol) IV over 1-2 min.<br>Seizure:<br>2 g 50% magnesium sulphate (4 ml; 8 mmol) IV over 10 min. |

**Table 13.1 Calcium (Ca$^{2+}$) and magnesium (Mg$^{2+}$) disorders with associated clinical presentation, ECG manifestations and recommended treatment**

**ALS**

# Poisoning

Poisoning is an infrequent cause of cardiac arrest, but remains a leading cause in victims younger than 40 years. It is also a common cause of non-traumatic coma in this age group.

Self-poisoning with therapeutic or recreational drugs is the main reason for hospital admission. Drug toxicity can also be caused by inappropriate dosing and drug interactions. Accidental poisoning is commonest in children. Homicidal poisoning is uncommon.

Industrial accidents, warfare or terrorism may cause chemical, biological, radiological or nuclear (CBRN) exposure. Decontamination and safe management for individual or mass casualty incidents is not part of this manual. Further information can be obtained from: www.ukresilience.info/

## Initial treatment

Supportive care based on the ABCDE approach to prevent cardiorespiratory arrest whilst awaiting drug elimination is the mainstay of treatment. Airway obstruction and respiratory arrest secondary to a decreased conscious level is common. Alcohol excess is often present with self-poisoning.

- After opening and clearing the airway, check for breathing and a pulse (if trained to do so). Avoid mouth-to-mouth ventilation in the presence of toxins such as cyanide, hydrogen sulphide, corrosives and organophosphates. Ventilate the patient's lungs using a pocket mask or bag-mask and the highest possible concentration of oxygen. In paraquat poisoning, lung injury may be exacerbated by high concentrations of oxygen; adjust the inspired oxygen concentration according to pulse oximetry or arterial blood gases.

- There is a high incidence of pulmonary aspiration of gastric contents after poisoning. In unconscious patients who cannot protect their airway, use a rapid sequence induction with cricoid pressure to intubate the trachea and decrease the risk of aspiration. This must be undertaken by persons trained in the technique.

- Provide standard basic and advanced life support if cardiac arrest occurs.

- Cardioversion is indicated for life-threatening tachyarrhythmias. Use the guidelines for peri-arrest arrhythmias (Chapter 12). Try to correct reversible causes.

- Drug-induced hypotension is common after self-poisoning. This usually responds to fluid therapy, but occasionally inotropic support is required.

- Once resuscitation is under way, try to identify the poison(s). Relatives, friends and ambulance crews can usually provide useful information. Patient examination may give diagnostic clues such as odours, needle puncture marks, pinpoint pupils, tablet residues, signs of corrosion in the mouth, or blisters associated with prolonged coma.

- Measure the patient's temperature – hypo- or hyperthermia may occur after drug overdose.

- Consult a regional or national poisons centre for information on treatment of the poisoned patient. In the UK, specialist advice about specific poisons can be obtained by accessing TOXBASE® (www.spib.axl.co.uk). Similar centres exist in other countries. The World Health Organisation lists poison centres (www.who.int/ipcs/).

## Specific treatments

There are few specific therapies for poisons that are useful immediately. The emphasis is on intensive supportive therapy, with correction of hypoxia, hypotension, acid/base, and electrolyte disorders.

Therapies include limiting absorption of ingested poisons, enhancing elimination, or the use of specific antidotes. Seek advice from a poisons centre for up to date guidance for severe or uncommon poisonings.

- Activated charcoal adsorbs certain drugs. Its value decreases over time after ingestion. Consider giving a single dose of activated charcoal to patients who have ingested a potentially toxic amount of poison (known to be adsorbed by activated charcoal) up to one hour previously. Give only to patients with an intact or protected airway. Multiple doses may be beneficial in life-threatening poisoning with carbemazepine, dapsone, phenobarbital, quinine and theophylline.

- Gastric lavage followed by activated charcoal therapy is useful only within 1 h of ingesting the poison. Generally, this should be carried out after tracheal intubation. Delayed gastric lavage has very little effect on drug absorption and may propel drugs further along the gastrointestinal tract.

- Whole-bowel irrigation can reduce drug absorption by cleansing the gastro-intestinal tract by enteral administration of a polyethylene glycol solution. Consider in potentially toxic ingestion of sustained release or enteric-coated drugs, oral iron poisoning, and the removal of ingested packets of illicit drugs.

- Urine alkalinisation (pH > 7.5) by giving IV sodium bicarbonate can be useful in moderate to severe salicylate poisoning in patients who do not need haemodialysis. Urine alkalinisation can also be useful in tricyclic overdose (see below).

- Consider haemodialysis for poisoning with methanol, ethylene glycol, salicylates, and lithium. Charcoal haemoperfusion may be indicated for intoxication with carbamazepine, phenobarbital, phenytoin, or theophylline.

- Specific antidotes include: N-acetylcysteine for paracetamol; high-dose atropine for organophosphate insecticides; sodium nitrite, sodium thiosulfate, hydroxocobalamin, amyl nitrite,or dicobalt edetate for cyanides; digoxin-specific Fab antibodies for digoxin; flumazenil for benzodiazepines; naloxone for opioids. Reversal of benzodiazepine intoxication with flumazenil is associated with significant toxicity in patients with benzodiazepine dependence or co-ingestion of proconvulsant medications such as tricyclic antidepressants. The routine use of flumazenil in the comatose overdose patient is not recommended.

## Specific antidotes

These guidelines address only some causes of cardiorespiratory arrest from poisoning.

### Opioid poisoning

Opioid poisoning causes respiratory depression, pinpoint pupils and coma followed by respiratory arrest. The opioid antagonist naloxone rapidly reverses these effects. There are fewer adverse events when the airway is opened and patients receive oxygen and ventilation (e.g., with pocket mask or bag-mask) before naloxone in opioid-induced respiratory depression; however, the use of naloxone may prevent the need for intubation.

The route for giving naloxone depends on the skills of the rescuer: intravenous (IV), intramuscular (IM), subcutaneous, endotracheal (ET) and intranasal (IN) routes can be used. The non-IV routes may be quicker because time is saved in not having to establish IV access, which can be extremely difficult in an IV drug abuser. The initial doses of naloxone are 400 mcg IV, 800 mcg IM, 800 mcg SC, 2 mg IN, and 1-2 mg ET. Large opioid overdoses require titration to a total naloxone dose of 6-10 mg. The duration of action of naloxone is 45-70 min, but respiratory depression may persist for 4-5 h after opioid overdose. Thus, the clinical effects of naloxone may not last as long as those of a significant opioid overdose. Give increments of naloxone until the victim is breathing adequately and has protective airway reflexes.

Acute withdrawal from opioids produces a state of sympathetic excess and may cause complications such as pulmonary oedema, ventricular arrhythmia, and severe agitation. Use naloxone reversal of opioid intoxication with caution in patients suspected of opioid dependence.

Cardiac arrest is usually secondary to a respiratory arrest and associated with severe brain hypoxia. Prognosis is poor. Giving naloxone is unlikely to be harmful. Once cardiac arrest has occurred, follow standard resuscitation guidelines.

### Tricyclic antidepressants

Self-poisoning with tricyclic antidepressants is common and can cause hypotension, seizures and arrhythmias. Most life-threatening problems occur within the first 6 h after ingestion. A widening QRS complex, increased QT interval and right axis deviation indicates a greater risk of arrhythmias and seizures (Figure 13.2). Sodium bicarbonate therapy aiming for an arterial pH of 7.45-7.55 may prevent these complications. Hypertonic saline may be an alternative to sodium bicarbonate.

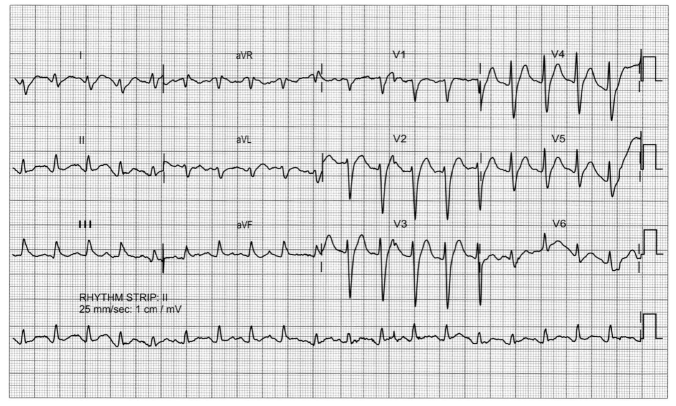

**Figure 13.2 12-lead ECG showing features of severe tricyclic antidepressant toxicity**

### Cocaine toxicity

Sympathetic overstimulation associated with cocaine toxicity may cause agitation, symptomatic tachycardia, hypertensive crisis, hyperthermia and myocardial ischaemia with angina. Small doses of intravenous benzodiazepines (midazolam, diazepam, lorazepam) are effective first-line drugs. Glyceryl trinitrate and phentolamine can reverse cocaine-induced coronary vasoconstriction; labetalol has no significant effect, and propranolol makes it worse. Use nitrates only as second-line therapy for myocardial ischaemia. Possible myocardial necrosis should be assessed using the ECG and cardiac markers (e.g., troponin) in patients with cocaine-related chest pain.

### Drug-induced severe bradycardia

Severe bradycardia from poisoning or drug overdose may be refractory to standard ALS protocols because of prolonged receptor binding or direct cellular toxicity. Atropine can be life-saving in organophosphate, carbamate or nerve agent poisoning. Give atropine for bradycardia caused by acetylcholinesterase-inhibiting substances. Large (2-4 mg) and repeated doses may be required to achieve a clinical effect. Isoprenaline may be useful at high doses in refractory bradycardia induced by beta-receptor blockade. Heart block and ventricular arrhythmias associated with digoxin or digitalis glycoside poisoning may be treated effectively with digoxin-specific antibody fragments.

Vasopressors, inotropes, calcium, glucagon, phosphodiesterase inhibitors and insulin-glucose may all be useful in beta-blocker and calcium channel blocker overdose. Transcutaneous pacing may be effective for severe bradycardia caused by poisoning and overdose (Chapters 11 and 12)

## Further treatment and prognosis

A long period of coma in a single position can cause pressure sores and rhabdomyolysis. Measure electrolytes (particularly potassium), blood glucose and arterial blood gas values. Monitor temperature because thermoregulation is impaired. Both hypothermia and hyperthermia (hyperpyrexia) can occur after overdose of some drugs. Retain samples of blood and urine for analysis. Be prepared to continue resuscitation for a prolonged period, particularly in young patients, as the poison may be metabolised or excreted during extended life support measures.

## Hypothermia

## Definition

Hypothermia exists when the body core temperature is below 35°C and is classified arbitrarily as mild (32-35°C), moderate (30-32°C), or severe (< 30°C). It can occur in people with normal thermoregulation who are exposed to cold environments, particularly wet or windy conditions, or following immersion in cold water. When thermoregulation is impaired, for example, in the elderly and very young, hypothermia may follow a mild cold insult. The risk of

hypothermia is also increased by drug or alcohol ingestion, illness, injury or neglect. Hypothermia may be suspected from the clinical history or a brief examination of a collapsed patient. A low-reading thermometer is needed to measure the core temperature and confirm the diagnosis.

## Decision to resuscitate

Hypothermia can exert a protective effect on the brain after cardiac arrest. Neurological recovery may be possible after hypothermic cardiac arrest, although those with non-asphyxial arrest have a better prognosis than those with asphyxial associated hypothermic arrest. Life-saving procedures should not be withheld on the basis of clinical presentation alone.

Beware of diagnosing death in a hypothermic patient, as hypothermia alone produces a very slow, small-volume, irregular pulse, and an unrecordable blood pressure. Hypothermia protects the brain and vital organs, and arrhythmias are potentially reversible either before or during rewarming. At 18°C, the brain can tolerate periods of circulatory arrest for ten times longer than at 37°C. Dilated pupils can be caused by a variety of insults and must not be taken as a sign of death.

On discovering a hypothermic cardiac arrest victim in a cold environment, it is not always easy to distinguish between primary and secondary hypothermia. Cardiac arrest could be due primarily to hypothermia, or secondary to a normothermic cardiac arrest (e.g., cardiac arrest caused by myocardial ischaemia in a person in a cold environment).

Do not confirm death until the patient has been rewarmed, or until attempts to raise the core temperature have failed; prolonged resuscitation may be necessary. In the pre-hospital setting, resuscitation should be withheld only if the patient has obvious lethal injuries or if the body is completely frozen making resuscitation attempts impossible. In the hospital setting use clinical judgment to determine when to stop resuscitating a hypothermic arrest patient.

## Treatment

The standard principles of prevention and life support apply to the hypothermic patient. Do not delay urgent procedures, such as intubation and insertion of vascular catheters.

- Open the airway and, if there is no spontaneous respiratory effort, ventilate the patient's lungs with high concentrations of oxygen. If possible, use warmed (40-46°C) and humidified oxygen. Consider careful tracheal intubation when indicated according to the ALS algorithm. Procedures can precipitate VF.

- Palpate a major artery and, if available, look at the ECG for up to 1 min and look for signs of life before concluding that there is no cardiac output. If a Doppler ultrasound probe is available use it to establish if there is peripheral blood flow. If the victim is pulseless, start chest compressions immediately. If you are not experienced in patient assessment or if there is any doubt about whether a pulse is present, start chest compressions until more experienced help is available. Both the respiratory rate and pulse may be very slow in severe hypothermia so more assessment time is necessary.

- Once resuscitation is under way, confirm hypothermia with a low-reading thermometer. Use oesophageal, bladder, rectal, or tympanic temperature measurements. Try to use a consistent method to allow serial comparisons of temperature.

- Use a 30:2 compression: ventilation ratio as for a normothermic patient. Hypothermia causes stiffness of the chest wall making ventilation and chest compression difficult.

- The hypothermic heart may be unresponsive to cardio-active drugs, attempted electrical pacing, and attempted defibrillation. Drug metabolism is slowed, leading to potentially toxic plasma concentrations of any drugs given repeatedly. Withhold adrenaline and other drugs until the patient has been warmed to a temperature greater than 30°C. Once 30°C has been reached, double the intervals between doses (twice as long as normal). As the patient's temperature returns towards normal (>35°C), use the standard drug protocols.

- Give drugs via a central or large proximal vein if possible.

- Remember to rule out other primary causes of cardiorespiratory arrest (e.g., drug overdose, hypothyroidism or trauma) or reversible causes using the four Hs and four Ts approach.

- Monitor electrolytes, glucose and blood gases regularly during resuscitation and post-resuscitation care as rapid changes can occur.

- Blood gas analysers will give blood gas values for a temperature of 37°C unless the patient's temperature is entered in to the analyser. Oxygen and carbon dioxide partial pressures are lower in hypothermia because gases become more soluble as blood temperature decreases. In clinical practice it is much easier to make all the measurements at 37°C. It is then only necessary to compare them with the well-known normal values for 37°C. This also enables comparison of serial results from blood gas samples taken during rewarming.

## Arrhythmias

As the body core temperature decreases, sinus bradycardia tends to give way to atrial fibrillation (AF) followed by ventricular fibrillation (VF) and finally, asystole. Follow standard treatment protocols.

- Arrhythmias other than VF tend to revert spontaneously as the core temperature increases and usually do not require immediate treatment. Bradycardia can be physiological in severe hypothermia. Cardiac pacing is not indicated unless the bradycardia persists after rewarming.

- If VF/VT is detected, give a shock; if VF/VT persists after three shocks, delay further defibrillation attempts until

the core temperature is above 30°C. Automated external defibrillators (AEDs) may be used on these patients.

## Rewarming

General measures for all patients include removal from the cold environment, prevention of further heat loss and rapid transfer to hospital. Rewarming may be passive external, active external, or active internal.

- Remove cold or wet clothing as soon as practical. Dry the patient, cover with blankets and keep them out of the wind.

- Warm passively with blankets and a warm room if the victim is conscious with mild hypothermia.

- In severe hypothermia or cardiac arrest, active warming is required. Forced air rewarming and warm IV fluids are effective in patients with severe hypothermia and a perfusing rhythm. Other warming techniques include the use of warm humidified gases and gastric, peritoneal, pleural, or bladder lavage with warm fluids (at 40°C), and extracorporeal blood warming with partial bypass.

- In the patient with cardiac arrest and hypothermia, cardiopulmonary bypass is the preferred method of active internal rewarming because it provides a circulation, oxygenation and ventilation while the core body temperature is increased gradually. Survivors in one case series had an average of 65 min of conventional CPR before starting cardiopulmonary bypass. Unfortunately, facilities for cardiopulmonary bypass are not widely available and a combination of other methods may have to be used.

- Do not over-warm the victim. In comatose survivors a period of therapeutic hypothermia may be beneficial (32-34°C). Hyperthermia is detrimental (see below).

- During rewarming, patients will require large volumes of fluids as their vascular space expands due to vasodilation. Warm all intravenous fluids. Use continuous haemodynamic monitoring and, if possible, treat the patient in a critical care unit.

## Post-resuscitation care

Avoid hyperthermia during and after the warming period. Once ROSC has been achieved, use standard strategies for post-resuscitation care, including mild hypothermia if appropriate (Chapter 14). There is no evidence for the routine use of steroids, barbiturates, or antibiotics.

## Hyperthermia

### Definition

Hyperthermia occurs when the body's ability to thermoregulate fails and core temperature exceeds that normally maintained by homeostatic mechanisms. Hyperthermia may be exogenous, caused by environmental conditions or secondary to endogenous heat production.

Environment-related hyperthermia occurs where heat, usually in the form of radiant energy, is absorbed by the body at a rate faster than can be lost by thermoregulatory mechanisms. Hyperthermia occurs along a continuum of heat-related conditions starting with heat stress, progressing to heat exhaustion, heat stroke and culminating in multi-organ dysfunction and cardiac arrest in some instances.

Malignant hyperthermia (MH) is a rare disorder of skeletal muscle calcium homeostasis characterised by muscle contracture and life-threatening hypermetabolic crisis following exposure of genetically predisposed individuals to halogenated anaesthetics and depolarising muscle relaxants.

## Heat stroke

Heat stroke is a systemic inflammatory response with a core temperature above 40.6°C accompanied by mental state change and varying levels of organ dysfunction. There are two forms of heat stroke: classic non-exertional heat stroke occurs during high environmental temperatures and often affects the elderly during heat waves; exertional heat stroke occurs during strenuous physical exercise in high environmental temperatures and/or high humidity and usually effects healthy young adults. Mortality from heat stroke ranges between 10-50%.

### Predisposing factors

The elderly are at increased risk for heat-related illness because of underlying illness, medication use, declining thermoregulatory mechanisms, and limited social support. There are several risk factors: lack of acclimatisation, dehydration, obesity, alcohol, cardiovascular disease, skin conditions (psoriasis, eczema, scleroderma, burn, cystic fibrosis) hyperthyroidism, phaeochromocytoma, and drugs (anticholinergics, diamorphine, cocaine, amphetamine, phenothiazines, sympathomimetics, calcium channel blockers, beta-blockers).

### Clinical Presentation

Heat stroke can resemble septic shock and may be caused by similar mechanisms. Features include:

- core temp 40.6°C or more;

- hot, dry skin (sweating is present in half cases of exertional heat stroke);

- early signs and symptoms include: extreme fatigue, headache, fainting, facial flushing, vomiting and diarrhoea;

- cardiovascular dysfunction including arrhythmias and hypotension;

- respiratory dysfunction including ARDS;

- central nervous system dysfunction including seizures and coma;

- liver and renal failure;

- coagulopathy;

- rhabdomyolysis.

Other clinical conditions need to be considered, including:

- drug toxicity;

- drug withdrawal syndrome;

- serotonin syndrome;

- neuroleptic malignant syndrome;

- sepsis;

- central nervous system infection;

- endocrine disorders e.g., thyroid storm, phaeochromocytoma.

## Treatment

The mainstay of treatment is supportive therapy based on optimising the ABCDEs and cooling the patient.

- Start cooling before the patient reaches hospital. Patients with severe heat stroke need to be managed in a critical care setting.

- Use haemodynamic monitoring to guide fluid therapy. Large volumes of fluid may be required. Correct electrolyte abnormalities.

- If cardiac arrest occurs, follow standard procedures for basic and advanced life support and cool the patient. Attempt defibrillation, if appropriate, according to current guidelines, while continuing to cool the patient.

- Provide post-resuscitation care according to normal guidelines (Chapter 14).

### Cooling techniques

Several cooling methods have been described but there are few formal trials on which method is best.

- Simple techniques include cool drinks, fanning the undressed patient and spraying tepid water on the patient. Ice packs over areas where there are large superficial blood vessels (axillae, groins, neck) are also useful. Surface cooling may cause shivering.

- In cooperative stable patients immersion in cold water is effective; however, this can cause peripheral vasoconstriction and reduce heat dissipation. Immersion is not practical in very sick patients.

- Use the same advanced cooling techniques as used for therapeutic hypothermia after cardiac arrest (see post-resuscitation care). Gastric, peritoneal, pleural or bladder lavage with cold water will decrease the core temperature. Consider the use of cold IV fluids, intravascular cooling catheters and extra corporeal circuits, e.g., continuous veno-veno haemofiltration or cardiopulmonary bypass.

- No specific drugs lower core temperature in heat stroke. There is no good evidence that antipyretics (e.g., NSAIDs or paracetamol) are effective in heat stroke.

## Malignant hyperthermia

Malignant hyperthermia is a life-threatening genetic sensitivity of skeletal muscles to volatile anaesthetics and depolarising neuromuscular blocking drugs occurring during or after anaesthesia. Stop triggering agents immediately; give oxygen, correct acidosis and electrolyte abnormalities. Start active cooling and give dantrolene.

# Drowning

Drowning is a common cause of accidental death. The most important detrimental consequence of drowning is hypoxia. Cardiac arrest is usually a secondary event. Prior alcohol intake is common amongst adult drowning victims. Immediate resuscitation at the scene is essential for survival and neurological recovery after drowning. This will require bystander provision of CPR plus immediate activation of the EMS system. Patients who have spontaneous circulation and breathing when they reach hospital usually recover with good outcomes. Remember, some patients may have had a primary cardiac arrest (e.g., caused by myocardial infarction whilst swimming).

## Definition

Drowning is defined as a process resulting in primary respiratory impairment from submersion/immersion in a liquid medium. Implicit in this definition is that a liquid/air interface is present at the entrance of the victim's airway, preventing the victim from breathing air. The victim may live or die after this process, but whatever the outcome, he or she has been involved in a drowning incident. Immersion means to be covered in water. For drowning to occur, usually at least the face and airway must be immersed. Submersion implies that the entire body, including the airway, is under the water or other fluid.

## Decision to resuscitate

Deciding whether to start or stop resuscitation of a drowning victim is notoriously difficult. No single factor predicts prognosis accurately.

- Start and continue resuscitation unless there is clear evidence that resuscitation attempts are futile (e.g., massive traumatic injuries, rigor mortis, putrefaction etc), or timely evacuation to a medical facility is not possible. Neurologically-intact survival has been reported in several victims submerged for greater than 60 min.

## Initial treatment

### Aquatic rescue and recovery from the water

- Ensure personal safety and minimise the danger to yourself at all times. If possible, attempt to save the drowning victim without entering the water. Talk to the victim, use a rescue aid (e.g., stick or clothing), or throw a rope or buoyant rescue aid if the victim is close to dry land. Alternatively, use a boat or other water vehicle to help with the rescue. Avoid entry into the water whenever possible. If entry into the water is essential, take a buoyant rescue aid or flotation device.

- Remove the victim from the water and start resuscitation as quickly and safely as possible. Cervical spine injury in drowning victims is uncommon (approximately 0.5%). Spinal immobilisation is difficult in the water and delays removal from the water and adequate resuscitation of the victim. Consider cervical spine immobilisation if there is a history of diving, water slide use, signs of severe injury, or signs of alcohol intoxication. Despite potential spinal injury, if the victim is pulseless and apnoeic remove them from the water as quickly as possible (even if a back support device is not available) whilst attempting to limit neck flexion and extension.

- Try to remove the victim from the water in a horizontal position to minimise the risks of post-immersion hypotension and cardiovascular collapse.

### Rescue breathing

- In the apnoeic victim, start rescue breathing as soon as the victim's airway can be opened and the rescuer's safety ensured. This can sometimes be achieved in shallow water. Mouth-to-nose ventilation can be used as an alternative to mouth-to-mouth ventilation if it is difficult to pinch the victim's nose. In deep water, start in-water rescue breathing only if trained to do so; ideally, with the support of a buoyant rescue aid. Do not try to resuscitate a victim in deep water unless you are trained to do so.

- If there is no spontaneous breathing after opening the airway, give rescue breaths for approximately 1 min (10 breaths). If the victim does not restart breathing, further management depends on the distance from land. If the rescuer and victim are close to land (< 5 min rescue time), if possible, continue rescue breaths whilst towing. If they are more than an estimated 5 min from land, give further rescue breaths over 1 min, then bring the victim to land as quickly as possible without further attempts at ventilation.

- There is no need to clear the airway of aspirated water. Remove debris manually or when dry land has been reached with suction if available. Most drowning victims aspirate small amounts of water, and this is absorbed rapidly into the central circulation. Do not use abdominal thrusts or tip the victim head down to remove water from the lungs or stomach.

### Chest compression

- As soon as the victim is removed from the water, check for breathing. If the victim is not breathing, start chest compressions immediately. Trained healthcare professionals can check for a pulse and other signs of life, but this may be even more difficult to find in a drowning victim, particularly if cold (see hypothermia). If there is any doubt about the diagnosis of cardiac arrest, start chest compressions. Chest compression is ineffective in the water.

**ALS**

### Defibrillation

If an AED is available, attach it to the victim and turn it on. Before attaching the AED pads, dry the victim's chest to enable adherence. Deliver shocks according to the AED prompts. If the victim is hypothermic with a core body temperature <30°C, limit defibrillation to a total of three attempts until the core body temperature rises above 30°C.

### Regurgitation during resuscitation

Regurgitation of stomach contents is common following resuscitation from drowning and makes airway management more difficult. If regurgitation occurs, turn the victim's mouth to the side and remove the regurgitated material using directed suction if possible. If spinal cord injury is suspected, log-roll the victim, keeping the head, neck, and torso aligned. Log rolling requires several rescuers.

## Advanced life support

### Airway and breathing

- Give high-flow oxygen if the patient is spontaneously breathing. Consider non-invasive ventilation or continuous positive airway pressure (CPAP) if the patient fails to respond to treatment with high flow oxygen. Use pulse oximetry and arterial blood gas analysis to titrate the inspired oxygen concentration.

- If initial measures fail and the patient is getting tired or has a reduced conscious level, consider early tracheal intubation and controlled ventilation. Use a rapid sequence induction technique for tracheal intubation.

- Protect the patient's airway in cardiopulmonary arrest early, ideally with a tracheal tube. Use a high inspired oxygen concentration during ventilation.

- Insert a nasogastric tube to decompress and empty the patient's stomach.

### Circulation and defibrillation

- Follow standard ALS protocols. If severe hypothermia is present (core body temperature <30°C), limit defibrillation attempts to three, and withhold intravenous drugs until the core body temperature increases above these levels. If moderate hypothermia is present, give intravenous drugs at longer than standard intervals (see hypothermia).

- During prolonged immersion, patients may become hypovolaemic from the hydrostatic pressure of the water on the body. Give intravenous fluid to correct the hypovolaemia but avoid excessive volumes, which may cause pulmonary oedema. After return of spontaneous circulation, use haemodynamic monitoring to guide fluid resuscitation.

## Post-resuscitation care

Follow the standard guidance for post-resuscitation care (Chapter 14).

- There are no important differences in the treatment of fresh- or salt-water drowning.

- Drowning patients have a high risk of developing the acute respiratory distress syndrome (ARDS) for up to 72 h after submersion. Tracheal intubation, sedation and controlled ventilation using lung-protecting strategies should be used.

- Pneumonia is common after drowning. Give antibiotics based on clinical assessment, results of cultures and advice from microbiologists.

- If submersion occurs in icy water (<5°C), hypothermia develops rapidly and can provide some protection against hypoxia. Hypothermia can also develop as a secondary complication of the submersion, and subsequent heat loss through evaporation, during attempted resuscitation. In these patients the hypothermia is not protective.

- In survivors who remain comatose, a period of therapeutic hypothermia (34°C) can be beneficial.

- Barbiturates, intracranial pressure (ICP) monitoring, and steroid do not alter outcome. A raised ICP usually indicates severe brain injury.

## Asthma

Asthma still causes many deaths in young adults, mostly among those with chronic severe asthma, adverse psychosocial circumstances and poor medical management.

It is important to recognise and treat exacerbations of asthma to prevent near-fatal asthma and cardiorespiratory arrest. National and international guidelines for the management of asthma exist (Figure 13.3). This manual will focus on the treatment of patients with near-fatal asthma and cardiac arrest.

## Causes of cardiac arrest

Cardiac arrest in the asthmatic is often a terminal event after a period of hypoxaemia; occasionally, it may be sudden. Cardiac arrest in asthmatics has been linked to:

- severe bronchospasm and mucous plugging leading to asphyxia;

- cardiac arrhythmias due to hypoxia, stimulant drugs (e.g., β-adrenergic agonists, aminophylline) or electrolyte abnormalities;

- dynamic hyperinflation can occur in mechanically-ventilated asthmatics. This is caused by gas-trapping in the lungs. The increase in intrathoracic pressure decreases cardiac output;

- tension pneumothorax (often bilateral).

The four Hs and four Ts approach to reversible causes will help identify these causes in cardiac arrest.

## Treatment

Use the ABCDE approach to assess severity and guide treatment.

ALS

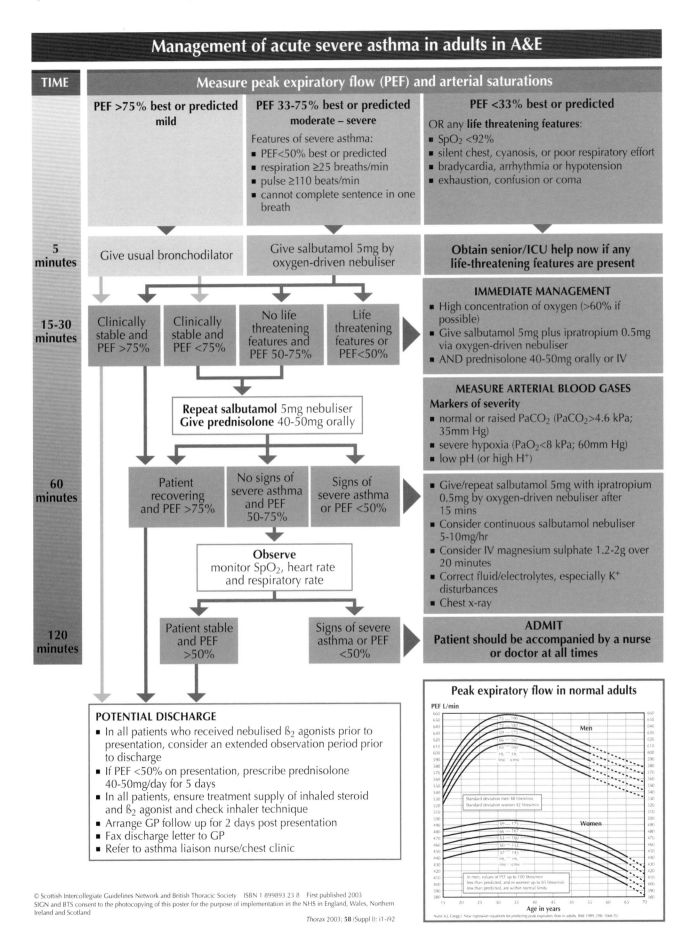

**Figure 13.3 SIGN and BTS guidelines for treatment of severe asthma**

Wheezing is a common physical finding, but severity does not correlate with the degree of airway obstruction. Other causes of wheezing include: pulmonary oedema, chronic obstructive pulmonary disease (COPD), pneumonia, anaphylaxis, pneumonia, foreign bodies, pulmonary embolism, bronchiectasis, subglottic mass.

The British Thoracic Society (BTS) and Scottish Intercollegiate Guidelines Network (SIGN) have published guidelines for the management of severe asthma (Figure 13.3). The severity of asthma is summarised in Table 13.2.

- The patient with acute severe asthma requires aggressive medical management to prevent deterioration. Experienced clinicians should treat these patients in a critical care area.

- Give oxygen to achieve an oxygen saturation ($SpO_2$) $\geq$ 92%.

- Salbutamol (5 mg nebulised) is the main therapy for acute asthma. Repeated doses every 15-20 min, or continuous doses, may be needed. Nebuliser units that can be driven by high-flow oxygen should be used. Remember that nebulised drugs will not be delivered to the lungs effectively if the patient is tired and hypoventilating.

- Give corticosteroids (prednisolone 30-40 mg orally or hydrocortisone 200 mg IV) early. Oral formulations have a longer half-life but the IV route is easier in near fatal asthma.

- Nebulised anticholinergics (ipratropium 0.5 mg 4-6 hourly) produce additional bronchodilation in severe asthma and in those who do not respond to ß-agonists.

- Magnesium sulphate (2 g IV slowly = 8 mmol) is also useful as a bronchodilator in severe or near-fatal asthma.

- Consider intravenous salbutamol in severe or near-fatal asthma. Intravenous salbutamol (250 mcg IV slowly) may provide additional benefit in those who are already receiving nebulised salbutamol. Use an infusion of 3-20 mcg min$^{-1}$ if necessary.

- Aminophylline should be considered only in severe or near-fatal asthma. A loading dose of 5 mg kg$^{-1}$ is given over 20-30 min (unless on maintenance therapy) followed by an infusion of 500-700 mcg kg$^{-1}$ h$^{-1}$. Addition of this drug to high doses of $\beta_2$-agonists increases side effects more than it increases bronchodilation. Check plasma theophylline levels repeatedly to avoid toxicity.

- These patients are often dehydrated or hypovolaemic and will benefit from fluid replacement.

- Helium/oxygen mixtures and intravenous ketamine do not have proven benefit. They should be considered only by those with expertise in their use.

- Mechanical ventilation is needed if the above therapies fail and the patient is becoming exhausted or comatose. Consider a trial of non-invasive face mask ventilation to prevent the need for tracheal intubation.

**Near-fatal asthma**
Raised $PaCO_2$ and/or requiring mechanical ventilation with raised inflation pressures

**Life-threatening asthma**
Any one of the following in a patient with severe asthma:

- peak expiratory flow (PEF) <33% best or predicted
- bradycardia
- $SpO_2$ < 92%
- dysrhythmia
- $PaO_2$ < 8 kPa
- hypotension
- normal $PaCO_2$ (4.6 - 6.0 kPa (35-45 mmHg))
- exhaustion
- silent chest
- confusion
- cyanosis
- coma
- feeble respiratory effort

**Acute severe asthma**
Any one of:

- PEF 33-50% best or predicted
- respiratory rate > 25 min$^{-1}$
- heart rate > 110 min$^{-1}$
- inability to complete sentences in one breath

**Table 13.2. The severity of asthma based on the BTS/SIGN guidelines**

## Cardiac arrest

- Give basic life support according to standard guidelines. Ventilation will be difficult because of increased airway resistance; try to prevent gastric inflation.

- Intubate the trachea early. There is a significant risk of gastric inflation and hypoventilation of the lungs when attempting to ventilate a severe asthmatic without a tracheal tube.

- The recommended respiratory rate (10 breaths min$^{-1}$) and tidal volume required for a normal chest rise during CPR should not cause dynamic hyperinflation of the lungs (gas trapping).

- If dynamic hyperinflation of the lungs is suspected during CPR, compression of the chest wall and/or a period of apnoea (disconnection of tracheal tube) may relieve gas-trapping. Although this procedure is supported by limited evidence, it is unlikely to be harmful in an otherwise desperate situation.

- Dynamic hyperinflation increases transthoracic impedance. In VF, consider higher shock energies for defibrillation if initial defibrillation attempts fail.

- Look for reversible causes using the 4 Hs and 4 Ts approach.

- Tension pneumothorax can be difficult to diagnose in cardiac arrest; it may be indicated by unilateral expansion of the chest wall, shifting of the trachea, and subcutaneous emphysema. Early needle decompression (thoracocentesis) followed by chest drain insertion is needed. In the ventilated patient, thoracostomy (a surgical hole in the chest wall and pleura) may be quicker to do and more effective for decompressing the chest (see trauma section).

- Always consider bilateral pneumothoraces in asthma-related cardiac arrest.

## Post-resuscitation care

- Follow standard guidelines for post-resuscitation care.

- Optimise the medical management of bronchospasm.

- Use permissive hypercapnia: it may not be possible to achieve normal oxygenation and ventilation in a patient with severe bronchospasm. Efforts to achieve normal arterial blood gas values may worsen lung injury. Mild hypoventilation reduces the risk of barotrauma and hypercapnia is typically well-tolerated. Target lower arterial blood oxygen saturations (e.g., 90%).

- Provide sedation (neuromuscular paralysis if needed) and controlled ventilation. Despite the absence of formal studies, ketamine and inhalational anaesthetics have bronchodilator properties that may be useful in the asthmatic patient who is difficult to ventilate.

- Involve a senior critical care doctor early.

# Anaphylaxis

Anaphylaxis is a rare, but potentially reversible, cause of cardiorespiratory arrest. Although the management of cardiac arrest secondary to anaphylaxis follows the general principles described elsewhere in these guidelines, the pathophysiological processes occurring during anaphylaxis require additional specific therapy.

Anaphylaxis is a severe life-threatening, generalised or systemic hypersensitivity reaction. Investigations will show whether the reaction is allergic (immunoglobulin E (IgE) or non IgE mediated) or non-allergic anaphylaxis. The term anaphylactoid reaction is no longer used.

## Aetiology

Although allergic reactions are relatively common, progression to a severe life-threatening reaction is rare. The commonest causes of life-threatening reactions are drugs, stinging insects and food. In as many as 5-20% of cases the trigger for the anaphylactic reaction cannot be identified.

- In hospital, neuromuscular blocking drugs (particularly suxamethonium), antibiotics, and intravenous contrast agents are the most common triggers for anaphylaxis.

- Outside hospital, aspirin, non-steroidal anti-inflammatory

drugs and antibiotics are the most common causes of drug-induced life-threatening anaphylaxis.

- Stings from insects belonging to the Hymenoptera order (e.g., hornets, wasps, honeybees, and fire ants) usually cause local reactions with pain and swelling at the site. Fatal anaphylaxis occurs in people who are re-stung after a prior sting has induced IgE antibodies. Fatal reactions occur within 10-15 min, with cardiovascular collapse being the commonest cause of death.

- Life-threatening allergic reactions to food are increasing. Nuts and seafood (in particular prawns and shellfish) are the most frequent triggers. Bronchospasm, angio-oedema, airway obstruction and asphyxia comprise the most frequent fatal mechanism.

- Latex, or natural rubber, is a significant trigger of anaphylaxis among hospitalised patients because of frequent instrumentation and operations in which latex products are used. Avoidance of latex containing products is the only effective therapy. Life-threatening anaphylactic reactions to latex are very rare.

## Recognition

An anaphylactic reaction is a severe, systemic allergic reaction characterized by multi-system involvement. It should be considered when two or more body systems are affected (cutaneous, respiratory, cardiovascular, neurological, or gastrointestinal), with or without cardiovascular or airway involvement

Early signs and symptoms can include urticaria, rhinitis, conjunctivitis, abdominal pain, vomiting, diarrhoea and a sense of impending doom. Flushing is common, but pallor may also occur. Marked upper airway (laryngeal) oedema and bronchospasm may develop, causing stridor and wheezing (or high airway pressures in ventilated patients). In asthmatics, this may be particularly severe and difficult to treat. Death can be from respiratory arrest caused by bronchospasm or upper airway occlusion, cardiogenic shock from the direct effect of anaphylactic mediators on the heart, or vasodilation causing relative hypovolaemia, exacerbated by true volume loss as increased capillary permeability results in extravasation of intravascular fluid.

Anaphylactic reactions vary in severity and progress may be rapid, slow, or (unusually) biphasic. Rarely, manifestations may be delayed (this may occur with latex allergy), or persist for more than 24 h.

The lack of any consistent clinical manifestation and a wide range of possible presentations can cause diagnostic difficulty. An alternative explanation for the 'reaction' is common. Clinical assessment helps make the diagnosis. The history of previous allergic reactions is important as well as that of the recent incident. Pay particular attention to the condition of the skin, the pulse rate, the blood pressure and the upper airways, and auscultate the chest. Measure and record peak flow where possible. Consider the diagnosis of other conditions only after anaphylaxis has been excluded; failure to identify and treat anaphylaxis can be fatal.

- ACE inhibitors can cause angio-oedema with marked swelling of the upper airway. This reaction may occur at any time and is not related to initial exposure to the drug. The swelling may not improve with adrenaline and best treatment for this form of angio-oedema is unclear. Early recognition, observation and appropriate airway management is critical.

- Hereditary angio-oedema is familial and indistinguishable from the early angio-oedema of anaphylaxis or drug-related angio-oedema. There is an absence of urticaria with hereditary angio-oedema. This is treated with C1 esterase inhibitor as a specific concentrate.

- Severe asthma presents with bronchospasm and stridor, which are also common features of severe anaphylaxis. Asthma attacks do not usually present with urticaria or angio-oedema.

- Rarely, panic attacks can be associated with functional stridor as a result of forced adduction of the vocal cords. As with asthma, there is usually no urticaria, angio-oedema, hypoxia or hypotension. Diagnostic difficulties arise as some patients may panic after onset of urticaria (e.g., latex contact), or become hypoxic after adducting their vocal cords.

- Vasovagal reactions (e.g., following an immunisation) can cause sudden collapse and extreme bradycardia that is mistaken for anaphylaxis. Recovery is usually relatively rapid after simple interventions (e.g., lying down) and is not associated with urticaria, angio-oedema or bronchospasm.

## Treatment (Figure 13.4)

- Recline the victim in a comfortable position. Lying flat, with or without leg elevation, may be helpful for hypotension but unhelpful for breathing difficulties.

- Remove the likely allergen (i.e., stop drug infusion or blood transfusion).

- Give high-flow oxygen (15 l min$^{-1}$).

- Give adrenaline intramuscularly to all patients with signs of shock, airway swelling, or definite breathing difficulty. Inspiratory stridor, wheeze, cyanosis, pronounced tachycardia, and decreased capillary filling indicate a severe reaction. For adults, give an intramuscular dose of 0.5 ml adrenaline 1:1000 solution (500 mcg). If there is no improvement repeat the dose after about 5 min. Several doses may be needed, particularly if improvement is transient. As an alpha-agonist, adrenaline reverses peripheral vasodilation and reduces oedema. Its beta-agonist properties dilate the airways, increase the force of myocardial contraction, and suppress histamine and leukotriene release.

- When given intramuscularly, adrenaline is very safe.

Adverse effects are extremely rare. Sometimes there has been uncertainty about whether complications (for example myocardial ischaemia) have been caused by the effects of the allergen or the adrenaline.

- Intravenous adrenaline (in a dilution of at least 1:10,000) is potentially hazardous and must be reserved for patients with profound shock that is immediately life-threatening and for special indications, for example during anaesthesia. A further ten-fold dilution to 1:100,000 adrenaline enables finer titration of the dose and increases its safety by reducing the risk of unwanted adverse effects. This should be carried out with, at least, electrocardiographic monitoring. Clinicians experienced in the use of intravenous adrenaline infusion may prefer to use the intravenous route in any patient with signs of severe anaphylaxis.

- Adrenaline may fail to reverse the clinical manifestations of anaphylaxis, especially in late reactions or in patients treated with beta blockers. Other measures then assume greater importance, particularly volume replacement.

- Give an H$_1$-antihistamine (e.g., chlorphenamine) 4 mg orally or 10-20 mg by slow intravenous injection. Consider also an H$_2$-blocker e.g., ranitidine (50 mg IV).

- Give corticosteroids after severe attacks, to help avert late sequelae. This is particularly important for asthmatics (who are at increased risk of severe or fatal anaphylaxis) if they have been treated with corticosteroids previously. Corticosteroids may help in the emergency treatment of an acute attack, and they also have a role in preventing or shortening protracted reactions.

- Nebulised salbutamol (5 mg repeated if necessary) can reverse refractory bronchospasm. Inhaled ipratropium (500 mcg, repeated as necessary) may be especially useful for treatment of bronchospasm in patients on b-blockers. Some cases of near-fatal asthma may really be anaphylaxis, resulting in mistaken over-treatment with conventional bronchodilators rather than more specific treatment with adrenaline. Consider the use of intravenous salbutamol, aminophylline or magnesium sulphate in severe bronchospasm (see asthma).

- If severe hypotension does not respond rapidly to drug treatment, give fluid; a rapid infusion of 1-2 litres may be required. Further fluid is likely to be required. Some patients may also require a continuous infusion of adrenaline for several hours.

- Other potential therapies to consider include:

  - Glucagon (1-2 mg every 5 min IM or IV) may be effective for patients unresponsive to adrenaline, especially in those receiving beta-blockers.

  - Immediately scrape away any insect parts at the site of the sting. Avoid squeezing.

ALS

## Anaphylactic Reactions: Treatment Algorithm for Adults by First Medical Responders

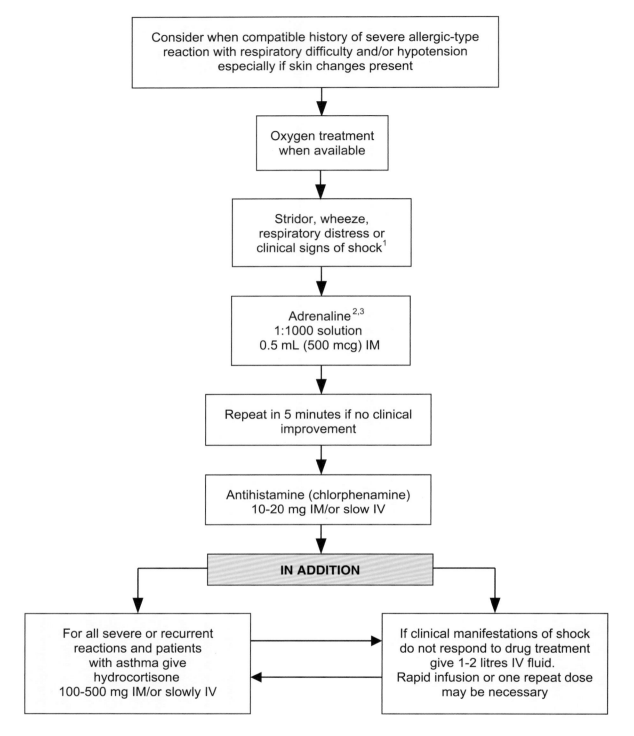

Consider when compatible history of severe allergic-type reaction with respiratory difficulty and/or hypotension especially if skin changes present

Oxygen treatment when available

Stridor, wheeze, respiratory distress or clinical signs of shock[1]

Adrenaline[2,3]
1:1000 solution
0.5 mL (500 mcg) IM

Repeat in 5 minutes if no clinical improvement

Antihistamine (chlorphenamine)
10-20 mg IM/or slow IV

**IN ADDITION**

For all severe or recurrent reactions and patients with asthma give hydrocortisone 100-500 mg IM/or slowly IV

If clinical manifestations of shock do not respond to drug treatment give 1-2 litres IV fluid. Rapid infusion or one repeat dose may be necessary

1. An inhaled beta$_2$-agonist such as salbutamol may be used as an adjunctive measure if bronchospasm is severe and does not respond rapidly to other treatment.

2. If profound shock judged **immediately** life threatening give CPR/ALS if necessary. Consider **slow** IV adrenaline 1:10,000 solution. This is **hazardous** and is recommended only for an experienced practitioner who can also obtain IV access without delay. Note the different strength of adrenaline that may be required for IV use.

3. If adults are treated with an adrenaline auto-injector, the 300 micrograms will usually be sufficient. A second dose may be required. Half doses of adrenaline may be safer for patients on amitriptyline, imipramine, or beta blocker.

**Figure 13.4 Anaphylaxis algorithm**

## Cardiac arrest

In addition to standard ALS, consider the following:

- Near-fatal anaphylaxis produces profound vasodilation and a relative hypovolaemia. Use at least two large-bore cannulae with pressure bags to give large volumes (as much as 4-8 l of intravenous fluid may be necessary in the immediate resuscitation period).

- Give an antihistamine intravenously if one has not already been given before the arrest.

- Steroids given during a cardiac arrest will have little immediate effect, but if ROSC is restored, they may be effective in the post-resuscitation period.

- Prolonged resuscitation may be required.

## Airway obstruction

- Airway obstruction may occur rapidly in severe anaphylaxis, particularly in patients with angio-oedema. Warning signs are swelling of the tongue and lips, hoarseness and oropharyngeal swelling.

- Consider early tracheal intubation; delay may make intubation extremely difficult. As airway obstruction progresses, both LMA and Combitube are likely to be difficult to insert. Attempts at tracheal intubation may exacerbate laryngeal oedema. Early involvement of a senior anaesthetist is mandatory when managing these patients.

- A surgical airway may be required if tracheal intubation is not possible.

## Observation

Warn patients with even moderate attacks of the possibility of an early recurrence of symptoms and in some circumstances keep them under observation for 8-24 h. This caution is particularly applicable to:

- severe reactions with slow onset caused by idiopathic anaphylaxis;

- reactions in severe asthmatics or with a severe asthmatic component;

- reactions with the possibility of continuing absorption of allergen;

- patients with a previous history of biphasic reactions.

## Investigations and further management

Measurement of mast cell tryptase may help with retrospective diagnosis of anaphylaxis. Take three 10 ml clotted blood samples:

- immediately after the reaction has been treated;
- about 1 h after the reaction;
- about 6 h and up to 24 h after the reaction.

Identification of the allergen after successful resuscitation from anaphylaxis is important to prevent recurrence. Refer the patient to a specialist clinic. Patients at very high risk of anaphylaxis may carry their own adrenaline syringe for self-administration and wear a MedicAlert bracelet. Report drug reactions to the appropriate monitoring agency.

## Cardiac arrest following cardiac surgery

After major cardiac surgery, cardiac arrest is relatively common, with a reported incidence of 0.7% in the first 24 h and 1.4 % within the first 8 days. Cardiac arrest is usually preceded by physiological deterioration, although it may occur suddenly in stable patients. Continuous monitoring on the intensive care unit (ICU) enables immediate intervention at the time of arrest. Survival to hospital discharge of patients having a cardiac arrest during the first 24 h after cardiac surgery is reported as 54-79% in adults and 41% in children.

## Aetiology

Perioperative myocardial infarction is the commonest cause of sudden cardiac arrest and is often secondary to graft occlusion. The main causes of cardiac arrest in the initial post-operative period are:

- myocardial ischaemia;

- tension pneumothorax;

- haemorrhage causing hypovolaemic shock;

- cardiac tamponade;

- disconnection of the pacing system in a pacing-dependent patient;

- electrolyte disturbances (particularly hypo/hyperkalaemia).

## Diagnosis

An immediate decision on the likely cause of cardiac arrest must be made to enable rapid intervention and successful resuscitation. Auscultation of the chest, examination of the ECG and chest radiograph, transoesophageal/transthoracic echocardiography and measurement of blood loss from chest drains help identify the cause of the arrest. Actively seek and exclude reversible causes of cardiac arrest: the 4 Hs and 4 Ts. Myocardial ischaemia often causes myocardial irritability and progressive hypotension before an arrest. A tension pneumothorax and cardiac tamponade will cause progressive hypotension and an increasing central venous pressure. Increasing airway pressures and poor air entry in the affected lung will differentiate between the two conditions. Lack of drainage of blood from the chest drains does not exclude haemorrhage or tamponade because drains may block with clot.

## Treatment

Follow the standard ALS protocols.

- Seek assistance from senior clinicians without delay.

- Exclude immediately correctable causes such as pacing lead disconnection and tension pneumothorax. Extreme bradycardia or asystole may respond to pacing via internal pacing wires (if present) connected to an external pacemaker.

- Ensure correction of hypo/hyperkalaemia and hypomagnesaemia. Rapid restoration of an adequate blood volume is important.

- Be careful when giving intravenous adrenaline as the resulting hypertension may cause catastrophic failure of anastomoses.

- Chest compression can cause sternal subluxation, fractured ribs and damage to grafts. Continuous observation of the invasive blood pressure will enable the force of compression to be optimised. Effective chest compression should take precedent over concerns about potential damage to grafts.

- Mechanical factors (e.g., haemorrhage, tamponade, graft occlusion) account for a substantial portion of causes of sudden cardiac arrest occurring in haemodynamically stable patients during the immediate post-operative period. Correction of these may require chest re-opening and therefore internal cardiac massage.

- Re-open the patient's chest immediately if there is no output with chest compression or if there is a shockable rhythm refractory to defibrillation. Management of asystole usually requires prompt chest opening. Opening of the chest is relatively straightforward and, if indicated, should be undertaken within 10 min of cardiac arrest.

- Consider training non-surgical medical staff to open the wound and remove sternal wires while a surgeon is summoned. Make sure that a chest-opening kit is immediately available on the ICU. Invasive blood pressure monitoring will guide the effectiveness of internal cardiac massage. Remove blood clot carefully, manually or by suctioning, to avoid damaging grafts. Early identification and treatment of underlying pathology is challenging under theses circumstances and requires an experienced surgeon.

- Consider emergency re-institution of cardiopulmonary bypass (CPB) to correct surgical bleeding or graft occlusion and rest an exhausted myocardium. Emergency institution of CPB should be available on all units undertaking cardiac surgery. Ensuring adequate re-anticoagulation prior to commencing CPB or the use of a heparin-bonded CPB circuit is important. The need for a further period of aortic cross clamping does not preclude a favourable outcome.

- Internal defibrillation with paddles applied directly across the ventricles requires considerably less energy than for external defibrillation. Biphasic shocks are more effective than monophasic shocks for direct defibrillation. For biphasic shocks, starting at 5 J optimises for lowest threshold and cumulative energy, whereas 10 or 20 J optimises for more rapid defibrillation and fewer shocks. Use double these energy levels for monophasic shocks.

## Trauma

Cardiac arrest secondary to traumatic injury has a very high mortality, with an overall survival of just 2.2% (range 0- 3.7%). In survivors, neurological disability is common. Cardiac arrest caused by blunt trauma has a very poor prognosis. Survival from cardiac arrest after penetrating trauma is slightly better.

Cardiac arrest from a primary medical problem (e.g., cardiac arrhythmia, hypoglycaemia, seizure) may cause a secondary traumatic event (e.g., fall, road traffic crash). Traumatic injuries may not be the primary cause of a cardiorespiratory arrest. Survival usually depends on early resuscitation by experienced rescuers.

Causes of cardiac arrest in trauma patients include: severe traumatic brain injury, hypovolaemia from massive blood loss, hypoxia from respiratory arrest, direct injury to vital organs and major vessels, tension pneumothorax, cardiac tamponade. There are no reliable predictors of survival for trauma-related cardiac arrest. The American College of Surgeons and the National Association of EMS physicians pre-hospital guidelines recommend withholding resuscitation in:

- blunt trauma patients presenting with apnoea, no pulse and no organised ECG activity;

- penetrating trauma patients found apnoeic and pulseless after rapid assessment for signs of life such as pupillary reflexes, spontaneous movement, or organised ECG activity.

## Treatment

- Use the ABCDE approach to assess and treat. Treatment on scene should focus on good-quality CPR and advanced life support and exclusion of reversible causes using the 4 Hs and 4 Ts.

- Undertake only essential life-saving interventions on scene and, if the patient has signs of life, transfer rapidly to the nearest appropriate hospital. Do not delay for spinal immobilisation.

- Effective airway management is essential to maintain oxygenation of the severely compromised trauma patient. Early tracheal intubation by experienced rescuers can be beneficial. Use basic airway management manoeuvres and alternative airways to maintain oxygenation if tracheal intubation cannot be accomplished immediately. If these measures fail, a surgical airway is indicated.

- Give a high concentration of inspired oxygen. Avoid excessive tidal volumes during ventilation.

- Start chest compressions if cardiac arrest is confirmed. In hypovolaemic cardiac arrest, or cardiac tamponade, chest compressions are less effective than normal.

- Decompress a tension pneumothorax quickly by lateral thoracostomy (incision in the lateral chest wall through to the pleural cavity). This is likely to be more effective than needle thoracostomy and quicker than inserting a chest tube.

- Bleeding must be stopped and blood volume restored as soon as possible. This may require direct pressure, splinting of fractures or immediate surgery.

- If available, ultrasound will help diagnose rapidly haemoperitoneum, haemo-or pneumothorax and cardiac tamponade. This requires a trained operator and should not delay treatments.

- Give intravenous fluids conservatively until bleeding is controlled. In the presence of uncontrolled bleeding, excessive fluid will increase the bleeding. The choice of fluid and blood products will depend on local practice.

### Emergency thoracotomy

- Consider on-scene resuscitative thoracotomy in cardiac arrest caused by penetrating chest trauma if it can be accomplished within 10 min after the loss of the pulse. This requires a trained rescuer.

- Consider emergency department thoracotomy (EDT):
  - After blunt trauma in patients with vital signs on arrival and a witnessed cardiac arrest.
  - After penetrating cardiac injuries in patients who arrive after a short on-scene and transport time with witnessed signs of life or ECG activity.
  - In penetrating non-cardiac thoracic injuries even though survival rates are low.
  - In patients with exsanguinating abdominal vascular injury even though survival rates are low. This procedure enables the thoracic aorta to be cross-clamped and should be used as an adjunct to definitive repair of abdominal vascular injury.
  - In trauma related cardiac tamponade, needle pericardiocentesis is probably not a useful procedure. It increases scene time, can cause myocardial injury and delays effective treatments such as emergency thoracotomy.

## Commotio cordis

Commotio cordis is actual or near cardiac arrest caused by a blunt impact to the chest wall over the heart. A blow to the chest during the vulnerable phase of the cardiac cycle can cause malignant arrhythmias (usually VF). Syncope after chest wall impact can be caused by non-sustained arrhythmic events. Commotio cordis occurs mostly during sports and recreational activities and victims are usually young males (mean age 14 years). Follow standard resuscitation guidelines.

## Pregnancy

The mother and fetus must be considered in emergencies during pregnancy. Effective resuscitation of the mother is often the best way to optimise fetal outcome.

Significant physiological changes occur during pregnancy; for example, cardiac output, blood volume, minute ventilation, and oxygen consumption all increase. The gravid uterus can cause compression of iliac and abdominal vessels when the mother is in the supine position, resulting in reduced cardiac output and hypotension.

## Causes of cardiac arrest in pregnancy

Cardiac arrest in pregnancy is most commonly caused by:

- pre-existing cardiac disease;
- thromboembolism;
- suicide;
- hypertensive disorders of pregnancy;
- sepsis;
- ectopic pregnancy;
- haemorrhage;
- amniotic fluid embolism.

Pregnant women can also have the same causes of cardiac arrest as females of the same age group (e.g., anaphylaxis, drug overdose, trauma).

## Treatment

- In an emergency, use the ABCDE approach. Many cardiovascular problems associated with pregnancy are caused by caval compression.

- To treat a distressed or compromised pregnant patient:
  - place the patient in the left lateral position or *manually and gently* displace the uterus to the left;
  - give 100% oxygen;
  - give a fluid bolus;
  - seek expert obstetric help immediately.

- In cardiac arrest, all the principles of basic and advanced life support apply.

- Summon help immediately. For effective resuscitation of mother and fetus, expert help must be obtained; this should include an obstetrician and neonatologist.

- Use a left lateral tilt of at least 15° to relieve caval compression. After 20 weeks gestation the pregnant woman's uterus can press down against the inferior vena cava and the aorta, impeding venous return and cardiac output. Caval compression limits the effectiveness of chest compressions.

ALS

- The method for tilting will depend on where the patient is and what is available. Improvisation will be needed. The patient's body will need to be supported on a firm surface to allow effective chest compressions. Methods for tilting include:

  - left lateral tilt if the victim is on a spine board or operating table;

  - sand bags, firm pillows, or a purpose made wedge (e.g., Cardiff Wedge) if available;

  - manual displacement of the uterus to the left;

  - using the thighs of kneeling rescuers to tilt the torso.

- A hand position higher than the normal position for chest compression may be needed to adjust for the elevation of the diaphragm and abdominal contents caused by the gravid uterus.

- There is an increased risk of pulmonary aspiration of gastric contents in pregnancy. Early tracheal intubation decreases this risk. Tracheal intubation can be more difficult in the pregnant patient. Expert help, a failed intubation drill, and the use of alternative airway devices may be needed.

- Attempt defibrillation using standard energy doses. Left lateral tilt and large breasts make it difficult to place an apical defibrillator paddle. Adhesive defibrillator pads are preferable to paddles in pregnancy.

## Reversible causes

Look for reversible causes using the 4 Hs and 4 Ts approach. Abdominal ultrasound by a skilled operator to detect possible causes during cardiac arrest can be useful; however, do not delay other treatments. Specific reversible causes of cardiac arrest in pregnancy are:

- **Haemorrhage:**  This can occur both antenatally and postnatally. Causes include ectopic pregnancy, placental abruption, placenta praevia and uterine rupture. Maternity units should have a massive haemorrhage protocol. Treatment is based on the ABCDE approach. The key step is to stop the bleeding. Consider the following: fluid resuscitation including use of a rapid transfusion system, correction of coagulopathy, oxytocin, ergometrine and prostaglandins to correct uterine atony, uterine compression sutures, radiological embolisation of a bleeding vessel, and surgical control including aortic cross clamping and hysterectomy.

- **Drugs:** Overdose can occur in women with eclampsia receiving magnesium sulphate, particularly if the patient becomes oliguric. Give calcium to treat magnesium toxicity (see life-threatening electrolyte abnormalities). Central neural blockade for analgesia or anaesthesia may cause problems due to sympathetic blockade (hypotension, bradycardia) or local anaesthetic toxicity.

- **Cardiovascular disease:** Pulmonary hypertension causes most deaths from congenital heart disease. Peripartum cardiomyopathy, myocardial infarction, and

aneurysm or dissection of the aorta or its branches, cause most deaths from acquired cardiac disease. Pregnant women with coronary disease may suffer an acute coronary syndrome.  Percutaneous coronary intervention is the reperfusion strategy of choice for ST-elevation myocardial infarction in pregnancy because thrombolytic therapy is relatively contraindicated.

- **Pre-eclampsia and eclampsia:** Eclampsia is defined as the development of convulsions and/or unexplained coma during pregnancy or postpartum in patients with signs and symptoms of pre-eclampsia. Magnesium sulphate treatment may prevent eclampsia developing in labour or immediately postpartum in women with pre-eclampsia.

- **Amniotic fluid embolism** can present with breathlessness, cyanosis, arrhythmias, hypotension, and haemorrhage associated with disseminated intravascular coagulopathy. Presentation is variable and may even resemble anaphylaxis. Treatment is supportive as there is no specific therapy.

## Emergency Caesarean section

When initial resuscitation attempts fail, delivery of the fetus may improve the chances of successful resuscitation of the mother and fetus. The best survival rate for infants over 24-25 weeks gestation occurs when delivery of the infant is achieved within 5 min after the mother's cardiac arrest. Delivery relieves caval compression and may improve the likelihood of resuscitating the mother. Delivery also enables access to the infant so that resuscitation of the newborn child can begin.

In the supine position, the gravid uterus begins to compromise blood flow in the inferior vena cava and abdominal aorta at approximately 20 weeks' gestation; however, fetal viability begins at approximately 24-25 weeks.

- **Gestational age < 20 weeks.**  Urgent Caesarean delivery need not be considered, because a gravid uterus of this size is unlikely to compromise maternal cardiac output.

- **Gestational age approximately 20-23 weeks.** Initiate emergency delivery to enable successful resuscitation of the mother, not survival of the delivered infant, which is unlikely at this gestational age.

- **Gestational age approximately > 23 weeks.** Initiate emergency delivery to help save the life of both the mother and the infant.

## Planning

Advanced life support in pregnancy requires co-ordination of maternal resuscitation, Caesarean delivery of the fetus, and newborn resuscitation within 5 min. To achieve this, units likely to deal with cardiac arrest in pregnancy should:

- have in place plans and equipment for resuscitation of both the pregnant patient and the newborn child;

- ensure early involvement of obstetric and neonatal teams;

- ensure regular training of staff in obstetric emergencies.

# Electrocution

Electrical injury is a relatively infrequent but potentially devastating multi-system injury with high morbidity and mortality. Most electrical injuries in adults occur in the workplace and are associated generally with high voltage, whereas children are at risk primarily at home, where the voltage is lower (220 V in Europe, Australia, Asia; 110 V in the USA and Canada). Electrocution from lightning strikes is rare, but causes about 1000 deaths worldwide each year.

Factors influencing the severity of electrical injury include whether the current is alternating (AC) or direct (DC), voltage, magnitude of energy delivered, resistance to current flow, pathway of current through the patient, and the area and duration of contact. Skin resistance is decreased by moisture, which increases the likelihood of injury. Electric current follows the path of least resistance; conductive neurovascular bundles within limbs are particularly prone to damage.

Contact with AC may cause tetanic contraction of skeletal muscle, which may prevent release from the source of electricity. Myocardial or respiratory failure may cause immediate death:

- **Respiratory arrest** may be caused by central respiratory depression or paralysis of the respiratory muscles.

- Current may precipitate **VF** if it traverses the myocardium during the vulnerable period (analogous to an R-on-T phenomenon). Electrical current may also cause myocardial ischaemia because of coronary artery spasm.

- **Asystole** may be primary, or secondary to asphyxia following respiratory arrest.

Current that traverses the myocardium is more likely to be fatal. A transthoracic (hand to hand) pathway is more likely to be fatal than a vertical (hand to foot) or straddle (foot to foot) pathway. There may be extensive tissue destruction along the current pathway.

Lightning strikes deliver as much as 300 kilovolts over a few milliseconds. Most of the current from a lightning strike passes over the surface of the body in a process called external flashover. Both industrial shocks and lightning strikes cause deep burns at the point of contact - in industry the points of contact are usually on the upper limbs, hands and wrists, whilst with lightning they are mostly on the head, neck and shoulders. Injury may also occur indirectly through ground current or current 'splashing' from a tree or other object that is hit by lightning. Explosive force generated by a lightning strike may cause blunt trauma.

The pattern and severity of injury from a lightning strike varies considerably. As with industrial and domestic electric shock, death is caused by cardiac or respiratory arrest. In those who survive the initial shock, extensive catecholamine release or autonomic stimulation may occur, causing hypertension, tachycardia, nonspecific ECG changes (including prolongation of the QT interval and transient T-wave inversion), and myocardial necrosis. Creatine kinase may be released from myocardial and skeletal muscle. Lightning also causes various central and peripheral neurological problems.

## Treatment

Ensure that any power source is switched off and do not approach the victim until it is safe. High voltage (above domestic mains) electricity can arc and conduct through the ground for up to a few metres around the victim. It is safe to approach and handle casualties after lightning strike, although it would be wise to move to a safer environment. Follow standard resuscitation guidelines.

- Airway management can be difficult if there are electrical burns around the face and neck. Intubate the trachea early in these cases as soft tissue oedema can cause subsequent airway obstruction. Consider cervical spine immobilisation. This should not delay airway management.

- Muscular paralysis, especially after high voltage, may persist for several hours; ventilatory support is required during this period.

- Ventricular fibrillation is the commonest initial arrhythmia after high voltage AC shock; treat with prompt attempted defibrillation. Asystole is more common after DC shock; use standard guidelines for treatment of this and of other arrhythmias.

- Remove smouldering clothing and shoes to prevent further thermal injury.

- Give fluids if there is significant tissue destruction. Maintain a good urine output to increase excretion of myoglobin, potassium and other products of tissue damage.

- Consider early surgical intervention in patients with severe thermal injuries.

- Conduct a thorough secondary survey to exclude traumatic injuries caused by tetanic muscular contraction or from the person being thrown by the force of the shock.

Electrocution can cause severe, deep soft tissue injury with relatively minor skin wounds because current tends to follow neurovascular bundles; look carefully for features of compartment syndrome, which will necessitate fasciotomy.

## Further treatment and prognosis

Immediate resuscitation in young victims of cardiac arrest due to electrocution can result in survival. Successful resuscitation has been reported after prolonged life support. All those who survive electrical injury should be monitored in hospital if they have a history of cardiorespiratory problems or have suffered:

- loss of consciousness;

- cardiac arrest;

ALS

- electrocardiographic abnormalities;

- soft tissue damage and burns.

Severe burns (thermal or electrical), myocardial necrosis, the extent of central nervous system injury, and secondary multiple system organ failure, determine the morbidity and long-term prognosis. There is no specific therapy for electrical injury, and the management is symptomatic. Prevention remains the best way to minimise the prevalence and severity of electrical injury.

## Key learning points

- The conditions described in this chapter account for a large proportion of cardiac arrests in younger patients.

- Use the ABCDE approach for early recognition and treatment.

## Further reading

Soar J, Deakin CD, Nolan JP, et al. European Resuscitation Council Guidelines for Resuscitation 2005. Section 7: Cardiac arrest in special circumstances. Resuscitation 2005;67 Suppl 1:S135-70.

International Liaison Committee on Resuscitation. 2005 International Consensus on Cardiopulmonary Resuscitation and Emergency Cardiovascular Care Science with Treatment Recommendations. Part 4. Advanced life support. Resuscitation 2005;67:213-47.

Mahoney B, Smith W, Lo D, Tsoi K, Tonelli M, Clase C. Emergency interventions for hyperkalaemia. Cochrane Database Syst Rev 2005:CD003235.

Proudfoot AT, Krenzelok EP, Vale JA. Position Paper on urine alkalinization. J Toxicol Clin Toxicol 2004;42:1-26.

Idris AH, Berg RA, Bierens J, et al. Recommended guidelines for uniform reporting of data from drowning: The "Utstein style". Resuscitation 2003;59:45-57.

Bouchama A, Knochel JP. Heat stroke. N Engl J Med 2002;346:1978-88.

Grogan H, Hopkins PM. Heat stroke: implications for critical care and anaesthesia. Br J Anaesth 2002;88:700-7.

BTS/SIGN. British Thoracic Society, Scottish Intercollegiate Guidelines Network (SIGN). British guideline on the management of asthma. Thorax 2003;58(Suppl I):i1–94.

Mertes PM, Laxenaire MC, Alla F. Anaphylactic and anaphylactoid reactions occurring during anesthesia in France in 1999-2000. Anesthesiology 2003;99:536-45.

Joint Working Party of the Association of Anaesthetists of Great Britain and Ireland and the British Society for Allergy and Clinical Immunology. Suspected anaphylactic reactions associated with anaesthesia. 3rd ed. London: The Association of Anaesthetists of Great Britain and Ireland and British Society for Allergy and Clinical Immunology; 2003.

Mackay JH, Powell SJ, Osgathorp J, Rozario CJ. Six-year prospective audit of chest reopening after cardiac arrest. Eur J Cardiothorac Surg 2002;22:421-5.

Pottle A, Bullock I, Thomas J, Scott L. Survival to discharge following Open Chest Cardiac Compression (OCCC). A 4-year retrospective audit in a cardiothoracic specialist centre - Royal Brompton and Harefield NHS Trust, United Kingdom. Resuscitation 2002;52:269-72.

Department of Health, Welsh Office, Scottish Office Department of Health, Department of Health and Social Services, Northern Ireland. Why mothers die. Report on confidential enquiries into maternal deaths in the United Kingdom, 2000-2002: London: The Stationery Office; 2004.

Boyd R, Teece S. Towards evidence based emergency medicine: best BETs from the Manchester Royal Infirmary. Perimortem caesarean section. Emerg Med J 2002;19:324-5.

Katz V, Balderston K, DeFreest M. Perimortem caesarean delivery. Were our assumptions correct? Am J Obstet Gynecol 2005;192:1916-20.

Zafren K, Durrer B, Herry JP, Brugger H. Lightning injuries: prevention and on-site treatment in mountains and remote areas. Official guidelines of the International Commission for Mountain Emergency Medicine and the Medical Commission of the International Mountaineering and Climbing Federation (ICAR and UIAA MEDCOM). Resuscitation 2005;65:369-72.

# Post-resuscitation Care

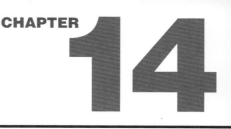

## CHAPTER 14

## Objectives

To understand:

▶ **The need for continued resuscitation after return of spontaneous circulation.**

▶ **The need for monitoring and investigations.**

▶ **How to facilitate transfer of the patient safely.**

▶ **How to ensure optimal organ function after cardiac arrest.**

▶ **The role and limitations of assessing prognosis after cardiac arrest.**

## Introduction

Return of a spontaneous circulation (ROSC) is an important step in the continuum of resuscitation. However, the next goal is to return the patient to a state of normal cerebral function, and to establish and maintain a stable cardiac rhythm and normal haemodynamic function. This requires further treatment, tailored to each patient's individual needs. The quality of treatment provided in this post-resuscitation phase significantly influences the patient's ultimate outcome. The importance of post-resuscitation care has been recognised by its inclusion as the new final ring in the revised Chain of Survival. The post-resuscitation phase starts at the location where ROSC is achieved but, once stabilised, the patient needs transfer to the most appropriate high-care area (e.g., intensive care unit (ICU), coronary care unit) for continued monitoring and treatment.

## Continued resuscitation

The ABCDE system-orientated approach to management should be followed in the immediate post-resuscitation phase pending transfer to an appropriate high-care area.

### Airway and breathing

Aim: to ensure a clear airway, adequate oxygenation and ventilation.

Patients who have had a brief period of cardiac arrest and have responded immediately to appropriate treatment (e.g., witnessed ventricular fibrillation (VF) reverting to sinus rhythm after early defibrillation) may achieve an immediate return of normal cerebral function. These patients do not require tracheal intubation and ventilation, but should be given oxygen by face mask. Hypoxia and hypercarbia both increase the likelihood of a further cardiac arrest and may contribute to secondary brain injury. Consider tracheal intubation, sedation and controlled ventilation for patients with obtunded cerebral function. After cardiac arrest,

hypocapnia induced by hyperventilation causes cerebral ischaemia. There are no data to support the targeting of a specific level of arterial $PCO_2$ after resuscitation from cardiac arrest, but it is reasonable to adjust ventilation to achieve normocapnia and monitor this using the end-tidal $CO_2$ and arterial blood gas values. Adjust the inspired oxygen concentrations to achieve adequate arterial oxygen saturation.

Examine the patient's chest and look for symmetrical chest movement. Listen to ensure that the breath sounds are equal on both sides. A tracheal tube that has been inserted too far will tend to go down the right main bronchus and fail to ventilate the left lung. If ribs have been fractured during chest compression there may be a pneumothorax (reduced or absent breath sounds) or a flail segment. Listen for evidence of pulmonary oedema or pulmonary aspiration of gastric contents. Insert a gastric tube - this will decompress the stomach following mouth-to-mouth or bag-mask ventilation, prevent splinting of the diaphragm, and enable drainage of gastric contents.

If the intubated patient regains consciousness soon after ROSC, and is breathing normally, consider immediate extubation: coughing on the tracheal tube will increase the patient's catecholamine levels significantly, which may provoke arrhythmias and/or hypertension. Ensure that a rigid sucker is available. Give the patient a high concentration of oxygen before and after extubation. If extubation is not possible sedate the patient to ensure the tracheal tube is tolerated, and provide ventilatory support.

## Circulation

Aim: the maintenance of normal sinus rhythm and a cardiac output adequate for perfusion of vital organs.

Cardiac rhythm and haemodynamic function are likely to be unstable following a cardiac arrest. Continuous monitoring of the ECG is essential. Seek evidence of poor cardiac function. Record the pulse and blood pressure and assess peripheral perfusion: warm, pink digits with a rapid capillary refill usually imply adequate perfusion. Grossly distended neck veins when the patient is semi-upright may indicate right ventricular failure, but in appropriate cases could indicate pericardial tamponade. Left ventricular failure may be indicated by fine inspiratory crackles heard on auscultation of the lung fields, and the production of pink frothy sputum. Try to optimise right and left heart filling pressures: measurement of central venous pressure will guide this. Once in a high-care area, the use of non-invasive cardiac output monitoring devices may be valuable. Infusion of fluids may be required to increase right heart filling pressures or conversely, diuretics and vasodilators may be needed to treat left ventricular failure. Early echocardiography is often helpful in guiding treatment.

Record a 12-lead ECG as soon as possible. Acute ST-segment elevation or new left bundle branch block in a patient with a typical history of acute myocardial infarction is an indication for treatment to try to re-open an occluded coronary artery (reperfusion therapy), either with thrombolytic therapy or by emergency percutaneous coronary intervention (PCI) (Chapter 3).

## Disability and exposure

Aim: to assess neurological function and ensure that cardiac arrest has not been associated with other medical or surgical conditions requiring immediate treatment.

Although cardiac arrest is frequently caused by primary cardiac disease, other precipitating conditions must be excluded, particularly in hospital patients (e.g., massive blood loss, respiratory failure). Assess the other body systems rapidly so that further resuscitation can be targeted at the patient's needs. To examine the patient properly full exposure of the body may be necessary.

Although it may not be of immediate significance to the patient's management, assess neurological function rapidly and record the Glasgow Coma Scale score (Table 14.1). The maximum score possible is 15; the minimum score possible is 3.

| Eye Opening | Spontaneously | 4 |
| | To speech | 3 |
| | To pain | 2 |
| | Nil | 1 |
| Verbal | Orientated | 5 |
| | Confused | 4 |
| | Inappropriate words | 3 |
| | Incomprehensible sounds | 2 |
| | Nil | 1 |
| Best Motor Response | Obeys commands | 6 |
| | Localises | 5 |
| | Normal flexion | 4 |
| | Abnormal flexion | 3 |
| | Extension | 2 |
| | Nil | 1 |

**Table 14.1 The Glasgow Coma Scale**

## Further Assessment

### History

Aim:  To establish the patient's state of health and regular drug therapy before the cardiac arrest.

Obtain a comprehensive history as quickly as possible. Those involved in caring for the patient immediately before the cardiac arrest may be able to help (e.g., emergency medical personnel, primary/community care physician, and relatives). Specifically, symptoms of cardiac disease should be sought. Consider other causes of cardiac arrest if there is little to

suggest primary cardiac disease (e.g., drug overdose, subarachnoid haemorrhage). Make a note of any delay before the start of resuscitation, and the duration of the resuscitation; this may have prognostic significance.

### Monitoring

Aim: to enable continuous assessment of vital organ function and to identify trends.

Continuous monitoring of ECG, arterial and possibly central venous blood pressures, respiratory rate, pulse oximetry, capnography, core temperature and urinary output is essential to detect changes during the period of instability that follows resuscitation from cardiac arrest. Monitor continuously the effects of medical interventions (e.g., assisted ventilation, diuretic therapy).

### Investigations

Several physiological variables may be abnormal immediately after a cardiac arrest and urgent biochemical and cardiological investigations should be undertaken (Table 14.2).

### Arterial blood gases

Guidance on the interpretation of arterial blood gas values is given at the end of this chapter.

Hypoperfusion during the period of cardiac arrest will usually cause a metabolic acidosis (increase in plasma hydrogen ion concentration). This will cause a low pH (acidaemia), low standard bicarbonate and a base deficit. The rate at which the acidaemia resolves in the post-resuscitation period is an important guide to the adequacy of tissue perfusion. The most effective way of correcting any acidaemia is by addressing the underlying cause. For example, poor peripheral perfusion is better treated by giving fluid and inotropic drugs than by giving alkali.

The normal physiological response to a metabolic acidosis is to reduce the $PaCO_2$ by an increase in ventilation (respiratory compensation). The patient who is breathing spontaneously may fail to achieve this if ventilation is depressed by sedatives, a reduced conscious level, or significant pulmonary disease. In these cases, the $PaCO_2$ may increase, causing a combined respiratory and metabolic acidosis and profound acidaemia.

Giving bicarbonate may, paradoxically, increase intracellular acidosis, as it is converted to carbon dioxide with the release of hydrogen ions within the cell. Indications for bicarbonate include cardiac arrest associated with hyperkalaemia or tricyclic overdose.

| FULL BLOOD COUNT |
|---|
| To exclude anaemia as contributor to myocardial ischaemia and provide baseline values. |
| **BIOCHEMISTRY** |
| To assess renal function.<br>To assess electrolyte concentrations ($K^+$, $Mg^{2+}$, and $Ca^{2+}$).*<br>To ensure normoglycaemia.<br>To commence serial cardiac troponin and enzyme. measurements.<br>To provide baseline values. |
| **12-LEAD ECG** |
| To record cardiac rhythm.**<br>To look for evidence of acute coronary syndrome.<br>To look for evidence of old myocardial infarction.<br>To provide a baseline record. |
| **CHEST RADIOGRAPH** |
| To establish the position of a tracheal tube, a gastric tube, and/or a central venous line.<br>To check for evidence of pulmonary oedema.<br>To check for evidence of pulmonary aspiration.<br>To exclude pneumothorax.<br>To assess cardiac contour (accurate assessment of heart size requires standard PA erect radiograph – not always practicable in the post-resuscitation situation). |
| **ARTERIAL BLOOD GAS** |
| To ensure adequacy of ventilation and oxygenation.<br>To ensure correction of acid/base imbalance. |
| **ECHOCARDIOGRAPHY** |
| In appropriate patients:<br>To identify contributing causes to cardiac arrest.<br>To assess LV and RV structure and function. |

*Immediately after a cardiac arrest there is typically a period of hyperkalaemia. However endogenous catecholamine release promotes influx of potassium into cells and may cause hypokalaemia. Hypokalaemia may cause ventricular arrhythmias. Give potassium to maintain the serum potassium between 4.0-4.5 mmol $l^{-1}$.

**Normal sinus rhythm is required for optimal cardiac function. Atrial contraction contributes significantly to ventricular filling, especially in the presence of myocardial disease and valve disease. Loss of the sequential atrial and ventricular contraction of sinus rhythm may reduce cardiac output substantially in some patients.

**Table 14.2 Investigations after restoration of circulation**

# Patient transfer

Aim: to transfer the patient safely between the site of resuscitation and a place of definitive care.

Following the period of initial post-resuscitation care and stabilisation, the patient will need to be transferred to an appropriate critical care environment (e.g., intensive care unit or coronary care unit). The decision to transfer a patient from the place where stabilisation has been achieved should be made only after discussion with senior members of the admitting team. Continue all established monitoring during the transfer and secure all cannulae, catheters, tubes and drains. Make a full re-assessment immediately before the patient is transferred. Ensure that portable suction apparatus, an oxygen supply and a defibrillator/ monitor accompany the patient and transfer team.

The transfer team should comprise individuals capable of monitoring the patient and responding appropriately to any change in patient condition, including a further cardiac arrest. The Intensive Care Society (UK) has published guidelines for the transport of the critically ill adult (www.ics.ac.uk). These outline the requirements for equipment and personnel when transferring critically ill patients.

# Optimising organ function

Aim: to optimise vital organ function and limit secondary organ damage.

The extent of secondary organ injury after ROSC depends on the ability of the heart and vascular system to deliver oxygenated blood. There are opportunities to limit the insult to organs following cardiac arrest.

## Heart and cardiovascular system

Haemodynamic instability is common after cardiac arrest and manifests as hypotension, low cardiac output and arrhythmias. This post-resuscitation myocardial dysfunction may be caused partly by reperfusion injury and is usually transient, often reversing within 24-48 h. The post-resuscitation period is associated with marked elevations in plasma cytokine concentrations, which manifests as a sepsis-like syndrome and multiple organ dysfunction.

In the ICU, an arterial line for continuous blood pressure monitoring is essential and the use of a non-invasive cardiac output monitor may be helpful. There are very few randomised trials evaluating the relationship of blood pressure to the outcome after cardiac arrest. In the absence of definitive data, target the mean arterial blood pressure to achieve an adequate urine output, taking into consideration the patient's usual blood pressure.

### Referral for implantable cardioverter defibrillator

Consider the possible requirement for an implantable cardioverter defibrillator (ICD) in any patient who has been resuscitated from cardiac arrest in a shockable rhythm

ALS

outside the context of proven acute ST segment elevation myocardial infarction. All such patients should be referred before discharge from hospital for assessment by a cardiologist with expertise in heart rhythm disorders (Chapter 11).

## Brain: optimising neurological recovery

### Cerebral perfusion

Immediately after ROSC there is a period of cerebral hyperaemia; however, after 15-30 min of reperfusion, global cerebral blood flow decreases and there is generalised hypoperfusion. Normal cerebral autoregulation is lost, leaving cerebral perfusion dependent on mean arterial pressure. Under these circumstances, hypotension will compromise cerebral blood flow severely and will compound any neurological injury. After ROSC aim to maintain mean arterial pressure at the patient's usual level.

### Sedation

Although it has been common practice to sedate and ventilate patients for up to 24 h after ROSC, there are no data to support a defined period of ventilation, sedation and neuromuscular blockade after cardiac arrest. The duration of sedation and ventilation may be influenced by the use of therapeutic hypothermia (see below). There are no data to indicate whether or not the choice of sedation influences outcome, but short acting drugs (e.g., propofol, alfentanil, remifentanil) will enable earlier neurological assessment.

### Control of seizures

Seizures and/or myoclonus occur in 5-15% of adult patients who achieve ROSC, and in approximately 40% of those who remain comatose. Seizures increase cerebral metabolism by up to four-fold. Prolonged seizure activity may cause cerebral injury, and should be controlled with benzodiazepines, phenytoin, propofol, or a barbiturate. Each of these drugs can cause hypotension and this must be treated appropriately. Seizures and myoclonus per se are not related significantly to outcome, but status epilepticus and, in particular, status myoclonus, are associated with a poor outcome.

### Temperature control

#### Treatment of hyperthermia

A period of hyperthermia is common in the first 48 h after cardiac arrest. The risk of a poor neurological outcome increases for each degree of body temperature over 37°C. Treat any hyperthermia occurring in the first 72 h after cardiac arrest with antipyretics or active cooling.

#### Therapeutic hypothermia

Mild hypothermia is thought to suppress many of the chemical reactions associated with reperfusion injury. These reactions include free radical production, excitatory amino acid release, and calcium shifts, which can in turn lead to mitochondrial damage and apoptosis (programmed cell death). Two randomised clinical trials showed improved outcome in adults remaining comatose after initial resuscitation from out-of-hospital VF cardiac arrest, who were cooled within minutes to hours after ROSC. These patients were cooled to 32-34°C for 12-24 h. One small study has shown benefit after therapeutic hypothermia in comatose survivors of non-VF arrest.

External and/or internal cooling techniques can be used to initiate cooling. An infusion of 30 ml kg$^{-1}$ of 4°C 0.9%. saline decreases core temperature by 1.5°C. Intravascular cooling using a purpose-made device incorporating temperature feedback enables more precise control of core temperature than external methods, but it is unknown whether this improves outcome.

Complications of mild therapeutic hypothermia include infection, cardiovascular instability, coagulopathy, hyperglycaemia, and electrolyte abnormalities such as hypophosphataemia and hypomagnesaemia.

Unconscious adult patients with spontaneous circulation after out-of-hospital VF cardiac arrest should be cooled to 32-34°C. Cooling should be started as soon as possible and continued for at least 12-24 h. Induced hypothermia might also benefit unconscious adult patients with spontaneous circulation after out-of-hospital cardiac arrest from a non-shockable rhythm, or cardiac arrest in hospital. Precisely which patients are cooled after cardiac arrest will be determined by local policy; however, generally recognised exclusion criteria include severe systemic infection, multiple organ failure, and severe cardiogenic shock. Treat shivering by ensuring adequate sedation and giving neuromuscular blocking drugs. Bolus doses of neuromuscular blockers are usually adequate but infusions are necessary occasionally. Re-warm the patient slowly (0.25-0.5°C h$^{-1}$) and avoid hyperthermia. The optimum target temperature, rate of cooling, duration of hypothermia, and rate of re-warming have yet to be determined.

### Other supportive therapies

#### Blood glucose control

There is a strong association between high blood glucose after resuscitation from cardiac arrest and poor neurological outcome. Tight control of blood glucose (4.4-6.1 mmol l$^{-1}$) using insulin reduces hospital mortality in critically ill adults, but this has not been demonstrated in post cardiac arrest patients specifically. The benefit is thought to result from the strict glycaemic control rather than the dose of insulin infused. There are no randomised controlled human trials of glucose control after cardiac arrest.

The optimal blood glucose target in critically ill patients has not been determined. Comatose patients are at particular risk from unrecognised hypoglycaemia and the risk of this complication occurring increases as the target blood glucose concentration is lowered.

In common with all critically ill patients, patients admitted to a critical care environment after cardiac arrest should have their blood glucose monitored frequently and hyperglycaemia treated with an insulin infusion. The blood glucose concentration that triggers insulin therapy and the target range of blood glucose concentrations should be determined by local policy.

## Prognostication

Aim: to predict at the earliest opportunity those patients who will not survive despite a return of spontaneous circulation

Of 22,105 patients admitted to intensive care units in the UK after cardiac arrest, 9,974 (45%) survived to leave intensive care and 6353 (30%) survived to hospital discharge [data from Intensive Care National Audit and Research Centre (ICNARC), London, December 1995 - October 2004]. Once a heart has been resuscitated to a stable rhythm and cardiac output, the organ that influences an individual's survival most significantly is the brain. Two thirds of those dying after admission to ICU following out-of-hospital cardiac arrest die from neurological injury. A quarter of those dying after admission to ICU following in-hospital cardiac arrest die from neurological injury.

A means of predicting neurological outcome that can be applied to individual patients immediately after ROSC is required. Such a test of prognosis must have 100% specificity; i.e., the test must not predict a poor outcome in a patient who then achieves an acceptable quality of life.

### Clinical tests

There are no neurological signs that can predict outcome in the first hours after ROSC. By three days after the onset of coma relating to cardiac arrest, 50% of patients with no chance of ultimate recovery have died. In the remaining patients, the absence of pupil light reflexes on day three and an absent motor response to pain on day three are independently predictive of a poor outcome (death or vegetative state) with very high specificity.

### Biochemical tests

Measurement of serum neuron specific enolase (NSE) and protein S-100b may be useful in determining the outcome of a cardiac arrest. However, the 95% confidence interval (CI) in the trials undertaken to date is wide and in many of the studies return to consciousness (without comment on level of function) was considered a 'good' outcome.

### Electrophysiological tests

Median nerve somatosensory evoked potentials in normothermic patients, comatose for at least 72 h after cardiac arrest, predict poor outcome with 100% specificity. Bilateral absence of the N20 component of the evoked potentials in comatose patients with coma of hypoxic-anoxic origin is uniformly fatal.

The electroencephalogram (EEG) provides limited prognostic information when it is recorded within 24-48 h after ROSC. A normal or grossly abnormal EEG predicts outcome reliably, but an EEG between these extremes is unreliable for prediction of prognosis.

## Care of the resuscitation team

Audit all resuscitation attempts and record the data using the standard Utstein template to enable comparison between different institutions (Chapter 17). Feedback for the resuscitation team should be constructive and not based on a fault/blame culture. Whether the resuscitation attempt was successful or not, the patient's relatives will require considerable support. Consider the pastoral needs of all those associated with the arrest.

## Acid–base balance: interpreting arterial blood gases

Unless a spontaneous circulation is restored very rapidly, cardiac arrest is associated with profound changes in acid base balance. In the immediate post resuscitation period, the ability to interpret the results of arterial blood analysis is important in determining the optimal treatment of the patient.

Enzymes within the cells of the body require a tightly controlled biochemical environment in order to function normally. The concentration of hydrogen ions ($H^+$) is low but crucial for normal enzyme function. The common ions in plasma, such as sodium and potassium, exist in concentrations of millimoles per litre (mmol $l^{-1}$) but the normal plasma concentration of $H^+$ is 40 nanomoles per litre (nmol $l^{-1}$). The $H^+$ concentration is most commonly represented as pH, which is the negative logarithm of the $H^+$ concentration. Thus, doubling or halving the $H^+$ concentration reduces or increases the pH by approximately 0.3 (Table 14.3). The normal extracellular pH is 7.35 – 7.45.

| pH | $H^+$ (nmol $l^{-1}$) |
|-----|-----|
| 6.8 | 160 |
| 7.1 | 80 |
| 7.4 | 40 |
| 7.7 | 20 |

**Table 14.3 The relationship between pH and H+ concentration**

### Definitions

| | |
|---|---|
| **Acid** | A proton donor or $H^+$ ion donor. |
| **Base** | A proton acceptor or $H^+$ ion acceptor. |
| **Acidaemia** | Blood pH < 7.35. |
| **Alkalaemia** | Blood pH > 7.45. |
| **Acidosis** | An abnormal process that tends to lower the blood pH. |
| **Alkalosis** | An abnormal process that tends to raise the blood pH. |
| **Mixed disorder** | Two or more primary acid-base abnormalities coexist. |

ALS

| | |
|---|---|
| **Compensation** | The normal body processes that returns blood pH to or towards normal (e.g., respiratory or renal). |
| **Buffer** | A substance that counteracts the effect on pH of an acid or base. |
| **FiO$_2$** | Fraction of inspired oxygen. At any altitude the FiO$_2$ of air is 0.21. This is often described as a percentage, e.g., 21%. |
| **PaO$_2$** | Partial pressure of oxygen in arterial blood. The PaO$_2$ does not reveal how much oxygen is in the blood, but only the pressure exerted by dissolved O$_2$ molecules against the measuring electrode. Normal PaO$_2$ is age-dependent; when breathing air, the normal PaO$_2$ is 12.5 – 13.0 kPa (95 – 100 mmHg) at the age of 20 years and approximately 10.8 kPa (80 mmHg) at 65 years. |
| **PaCO$_2$** | Partial pressure of carbon dioxide in arterial blood (normal value 5.3 kPa [range 4.7 – 6.0] or 40 mmHg [range 35 – 45]). |
| **HCO$_3^-$** | Bicarbonate concentration (normal value 24 mmol l$^{-1}$ [range 22 – 26]). |
| **BE** | Base excess – the quantity of strong acid or base required to restore pH to 7.4. The normal range is plus 2 mmol l$^{-1}$ to minus 2 mmol l$^{-1}$. A positive value of BE indicates an excess of base (or deficit of acid), while a negative value indicates a deficit of base (or excess of acid). |

**An example of a 'normal' arterial blood gas analysis from a 70 year old patient is:**

| | |
|---|---|
| **FiO$_2$** | 0.21 (air) |
| **pH** | 7.39 |
| **PaCO$_2$** | 5.2 kPa (39.2 mmHg) |
| **PaO$_2$** | 11.2 kPa (85 mmHg) |
| **HCO$_3^-$** | 24 mmol l$^{-1}$ |
| **BE** | -0.5 |

## Oxygenation

The upper limit of the arterial PO$_2$ (PaO$_2$) is dependent on the alveolar PO$_2$ (PAO$_2$). The arterial PO$_2$ is always lower than the alveolar PO$_2$ and the extent of this alveolar-arterial gap is increased in the presence of lung disease (poorly functioning lungs reduce the passage of oxygen from the alveoli to the pulmonary blood). Simplistically, the difference between the PO$_2$ in the inspired gas at the mouth and the arterial PO$_2$ is roughly 10 kPa in a healthy person. At sea level, 1% O$_2$ is approximately 1 kPa. Thus, when

breathing 21% oxygen, a person with normal lungs should have an arterial PO$_2$ of greater than 11 kPa (80 mmHg) (i.e., 21-10 kPa = 11 kPa). Breathing 50% oxygen at sea level in the absence of pulmonary disease will result in an arterial PO$_2$ of about 40 kPa (300 mmHg) (i.e., 50-10 kPa = 40 kPa).

Restoring adequate tissue oxygenation is fundamental to resuscitation. Hypoxaemia must be treated by increasing the FiO$_2$ and by ensuring a patent airway and adequate ventilation. Aim to achieve an oxygen saturation of at least 92% (equating to a PaO$_2$ of 8-9 kPa). Some patients, such as those with chronic obstructive pulmonary disease or those undergoing prolonged mechanical ventilation on ICU, may be treated more appropriately with lower oxygen saturations (88-89%).

In the presence of supplementary oxygen, a 'normal' PaO$_2$ does not necessarily indicate adequate ventilation. Even small increases in FiO$_2$ will overcome any hypoxaemia caused by high alveolar PCO$_2$ (hypoventilation).

The relationship between the partial pressure of oxygen and the percentage saturation of haemoglobin with oxygen (SaO$_2$) is described by the oxyhaemoglobin dissociation curve (Figure 14.1). This curve is sigmoid shaped. The flat upper part of the curve means that as the PaO$_2$ falls, the SaO$_2$ is well maintained down to a PaO$_2$ of approximately 8 kPa, when the SaO$_2$ is about 90%. As the PaO$_2$ falls below this level, the SaO$_2$ falls precipitously.

## Buffering

The major body buffer systems involve bicarbonate, protein, haemoglobin and phosphate. The bicarbonate buffer system is the most important and is represented by the Henderson-Hasselbalch equation:

$$pH = 6.1 + \log \frac{[HCO_3^-]}{PaCO_2 \times 0.03}$$

(0.03 = solubility coefficient of carbon dioxide, mmol/mmHg)

## Respiratory and renal compensation

From the Henderson – Hasselbalch equation it is clear that an increase in PaCO$_2$ leads to a decrease in pH and a decrease in PaCO$_2$ leads to a rise in pH. Thus, the respiratory system is able to regulate pH. If the metabolic production of CO$_2$ remains constant, the only factor that affects PaCO$_2$ is alveolar ventilation. **An increase in alveolar ventilation will decrease the PaCO$_2$ and a decrease in alveolar ventilation will increase the PaCO$_2$.** The respiratory centre in the brainstem is sensitive to H$^+$ concentration and changes alveolar ventilation accordingly. For example, if the pH decreases, under normal circumstances an increase in ventilation would return the pH to normal. This process occurs within a few minutes.

ALS

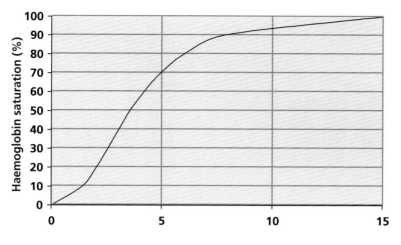

**Figure 14.1 Oxygen dissociation curve**

| Acid-base disorder | pH | PaCO₂ | HCO₃⁻ |
|---|---|---|---|
| **Respiratory acidosis** | ↓ | ↑ | N |
| **Metabolic acidosis** | ↓ | N | ↓ |
| Respiratory alkalosis | ↑ | ↓ | N |
| Metabolic alkalosis | ↑ | N | ↑ |
| **Respiratory acidosis with renal compensation** | ↓* | ↑ | ↑ |
| **Metabolic acidosis with respiratory compensation** | ↓* | ↓ | ↓ |
| Respiratory alkalosis with renal compensation | ↑* | ↓ | ↓ |
| Metabolic alkalosis with respiratory compensation | ↑* | ↑ | ↑ |
| **Mixed metabolic and respiratory acidosis** | ↓ | ↑ | ↓ |
| Mixed metabolic and respiratory alkalosis | ↑ | ↓ | ↑ |

\* If the compensation is virtually complete the pH may be in the normal range

– over compensation does not occur

Those marked in bold are particularly common after cardiac arrest

**Table 14.4 Summary of changes in pH, PaCO₂ and HCO₃⁻ in acid-base disorders**

The kidneys control acid base balance by controlling the secretion of H+ relative to the amount of filtered $HCO_3^-$. Hence the kidneys excrete either acid or alkaline urine. The renal response is slow and the maximum excretory capacity for H+ can be achieved only after several days.

## Classification of an acid-base defect

The primary defect in an acid-base disorder is defined by its initiating process, which can be metabolic (changes in $HCO_3^-$) or respiratory (changes in $PaCO_2$). A compensatory response describes the secondary physiological response to the primary disturbance. Over-compensation does not occur.

|  | Acidosis | Alkalosis |
|---|---|---|
| Respiratory | $CO_2$ ↑ | $CO_2$ ↓ |
| Metabolic | $HCO_3^-$ or base excess ↓ | $HCO_3^-$ or base excess ↑ |

When evaluated respiratory and acid-base disorders, the clinical features and plasma electrolytes must be considered together with the blood gases.

## The 5-step approach to interpretation of blood-gas values

1. Assess oxygenation

    Is the patient hypoxic?

    Is there a significant alveolar-arterial gradient?

2. Determine status of the pH or H+ concentration

    pH > 7.45 (H+ < 35 nmol l[-1]) – alkalaemia

    pH < 7.35 (H+ > 45 nmol l[-1]) – acidaemia

3. Determine respiratory component

    $PaCO_2$    > 6.0 kPa (45 mmHg) – respiratory acidosis (or respiratory compensation for a metabolic alkalosis)

    < 4.7 kPa (35 mmHg) – respiratory alkalosis (or respiratory compensation for a metabolic acidosis)

4. Determine metabolic component

    $HCO_3^-$    < 22 mmol l[-1] – metabolic acidosis (or renal compensation for a respiratory alkalosis)

    $HCO_3^-$    > 26 mmol l[-1] – metabolic alkalosis (or renal compensation for a respiratory acidosis)

    Some clinicians prefer to use the base excess (or deficit) instead of the $HCO_3^-$. As the changes in these values usually mirror each other, it makes no significant difference to the interpretation of the clinical condition. The normal base excess is +/- 2 mmol l[-1].

5. Combine the information from 2, 3 and 4 and determine which the primary disturbance is and whether there is any metabolic or respiratory compensation. In the presence of a low pH (acidaemia),

a high $PaCO_2$ implies a primary respiratory acidosis, while a low $PaCO_2$ implies respiratory compensation for a primary metabolic acidosis. In the presence of a high pH (alkalaemia), a low $PaCO_2$ implies a primary respiratory alkalosis, while a high $PaCO_2$ implies respiratory compensation for a primary metabolic alkalosis. It is also possible to have mixed acid base disorders, e.g., a combination of a respiratory and a metabolic acidosis creating an acidaemia or a combination of a respiratory and metabolic alkalosis creating an alkalaemia (Table 14.4).

## Key learning points

- After cardiac arrest, return of spontaneous circulation is just the first stage in a continuum of resuscitation.

- The quality of post-resuscitation care will influence significantly the patient's final outcome.

- These patients require appropriate monitoring, safe transfer to a critical care environment, and continued organ support.

- Our ability to predict the final neurological outcome for those patients remaining comatose after cardiopulmonary resuscitation remains very poor.

## Further reading

Bernard SA, Gray TW, Buist MD, et al. Treatment of comatose survivors of out-of-hospital cardiac arrest with induced hypothermia. N Engl J Med 2002; 346:557-63.

Hypothermia After Cardiac Arrest Study Group. Mild therapeutic hypothermia to improve the neurologic outcome after cardiac arrest. N Engl J Med 2002; 346:549-56.

Langhelle A, Nolan J, Herlitz J, et al. Recommended guidelines for reviewing, reporting, and conducting research on post-resuscitation care: The Utstein style. Resuscitation 2005;66:271-83.

Laver S, Farrow C, Turner D, Nolan J. Mode of death after admission to an intensive care unit following cardiac arrest. Intensive Care Med 2004;30: 2126-8.

Nolan JP, Morley PT, Vanden Hoek TL, Hickey RW. Therapeutic hypothermia after cardiac arrest. An advisory statement by the Advanced Life Support Task Force of the International Liaison Committee on Resuscitation. Resuscitation 2003;57:231-5.

Polderman KH. Application of therapeutic hypothermia in the intensive care unit. Opportunities and pitfalls of a promising treatment modality-Part 2: Practical aspects and side effects. Intensive Care Med 2004;30:757-69.

van den Berghe G, Wouters P, Weekers F, et al. Intensive insulin therapy in the critically ill patients. N Engl J Med 2001;345:1359-67.

Zandbergen EG, de Haan RJ, Hijdra A. Systematic review of prediction of poor outcome in anoxic-ischaemic coma with biochemical markers of brain damage. Intensive Care Med 2001;27:1661-7.

# Ethical Aspects of Resuscitation

 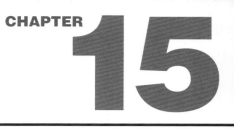

Throughout this chapter the term 'relatives' includes close friend/significant other.

## Introduction

Successful resuscitation attempts have brought extended, useful and precious life to many individuals. However, rates of survival and complete physiological recovery following cardiac arrest are poor. There are occasions when resuscitation attempts have merely prolonged suffering and the process of dying; in some cases resuscitation has left the patient in a persistent vegetative state. It is not an appropriate goal of medicine to prolong life at all costs.

Decisions about attempting resuscitation raise sensitive and potentially distressing issues for patients and relatives. These decisions may be influenced by individual, international and local cultural, legal, ethical, traditional, religious, social and economic factors. Some mentally competent patients decide they do not want treatment and express their wishes in an advance directive or living will. Therefore it is important that healthcare professionals understand the principles involved before they are put in a situation where a resuscitation decision must be made.

Discussion of the legal status of those who attempt resuscitation is not included in this chapter. Information on this topic can be found at www.resus.org.uk.

## Principles

The four key ethical principles are beneficence, non-maleficence, justice and autonomy.

**Beneficence** implies that healthcare professionals must provide benefit while balancing benefit and risks. Commonly this will involve attempting resuscitation but on occasion it will mean withholding cardiopulmonary resuscitation. Beneficence may also include responding to the overall needs of the community, such as establishing a programme of public access to defibrillation.

**Non-maleficence** means doing no harm. Resuscitation

should not be attempted in futile cases, and should not be attempted when it is against the wishes of a competent patient.

**Justice** implies a duty to spread benefits and risks equally within a society. If resuscitation is provided, it should be made available to all who will benefit from it within the available resources.

**Autonomy** relates to the patients making their own informed decisions rather than the medical or nursing professions making the decisions for them. This principle has been introduced particularly during the past 30 years arising from legislature such as the Helsinki Declaration of Human Rights and its subsequent modifications and amendments. Autonomy requires that the patient is adequately informed, competent, free from undue pressure, and that there is consistency in the patient's preferences.

## Advance directives

Advance directives have been introduced in many countries and emphasise the importance of patient autonomy. Resuscitation must not be attempted if CPR is contrary to the recorded sustained wishes of an adult who was mentally competent and aware of the implications at the time of making that advance decision.

The term advance directive applies to any expression of patient preferences. Refusal does not have to be in writing in order to be valid. If patients have expressed clear and consistent refusal verbally, this is likely to have the same status as a written advance directive. Patients should ensure that the healthcare team and his or her relatives are aware of their wishes if they are to be implemented.

In sudden out-of-hospital cardiac arrest those attending usually do not know the patient's situation and wishes, and an advance directive is often not readily available. In these circumstances resuscitation is begun immediately and questions addressed later. There is no ethical difficulty in stopping the resuscitation attempt that has started if the healthcare professionals are later presented with a valid advance directive limiting care.

There is still considerable international variation in the medical attitude to written advance directives. In some countries, such as the UK, the written advanced directive is legally binding. Where no explicit advance directive has been made and the express wishes of the patient are unknown there should be a presumption that healthcare professionals will, if appropriate, make all reasonable efforts to resuscitate the patient.

# When to withhold a resuscitation attempt

While patients have a right to refuse treatment, they do not have an automatic right to demand treatment; they cannot insist that resuscitation must be attempted in any circumstance. Doctors cannot be required to give treatment contrary to their clinical judgement. This decision is often complex and should be undertaken by senior, experienced members of the medical team.

The decision to withhold a resuscitation attempt raises several ethical and moral questions. What constitutes futility? What exactly is being withheld? Who should decide and who should be consulted? Who should be informed?

## What constitutes futility?

Futility exists if resuscitation will be of no benefit in terms of prolonging life of acceptable quality. Although predictors of non-survival after attempted resuscitation have been published, none has sufficient predictive value when applied to an independent validation group. Furthermore, the outcome for a cohort undergoing attempted resuscitation is dependent on system factors such as time to CPR and time to defibrillation. It is difficult to predict how these factors will impact on the outcome of individuals.

Inevitably, judgements will have to be made, and there will be grey areas where subjective opinions are required in patients with comorbidity such as heart failure, chronic respiratory disease, asphyxia, major trauma, head injury and neurological disease. The age of the patient may feature in the decision but is only a relatively weak independent predictor of outcome; however, the elderly commonly have significant comorbidity, which influences outcome.

## What exactly should be withheld?

Do not attempt resuscitation (DNAR) means that in the event of cardiac or respiratory arrest CPR, should not be started — nothing more than that. Other treatment should be continued, especially pain relief and sedation, as required. Also, treatment such as ventilation and oxygen therapy, nutrition, antibiotics, fluid and vasopressors, is continued as indicated, if it is considered to be contributing to the quality of life. If not, orders not to continue or initiate any such treatments should be made independently of DNAR orders.

While DNAR orders for many years in many countries were written by single doctors, often without consulting the patient, relatives or other health personnel, there are now clear procedural requirements or guidelines in many countries.

## Who should decide not to attempt resuscitation and who should be consulted?

The overall responsibility for this decision rests with the senior hospital doctor or primary care doctor in charge of the patient after appropriate consultation with other healthcare professionals involved in the patient's care. People have ethical and legal rights to be involved in decisions that relate to them and this should be discussed with the patient. It is good practice to involve relatives in decisions although they have no legal status in terms of actual decision-making. If the patient is competent his or her agreement should be sought. Refusal from a competent patient to allow information to be disclosed to relatives should be respected. Ideally, decisions should be made in advance.

Decisions by legal authorities are fraught with delays and uncertainties, especially if there is an adversarial legal system, and should be sought only if there are irreconcilable differences between the parties involved. In especially difficult cases, the senior doctor may wish to consult his/her own medical defence society for a legal opinion.

## Who should be informed?

Once the decision has been made it must be communicated clearly to all who may be involved, including the patient. Unless the patient refuses, the decision should also be communicated to the patient's relatives. The decision, the reasons for it, and a record of who has been involved in the discussions should be recorded in the medical notes — ideally on a special DNAR form — and should clearly document the date the decision was made. The decision should be recorded in the nursing records. The decision must be communicated to all those involved in the patient's care.

# When to abandon the resuscitation attempt

The majority of resuscitation attempts do not succeed and have to be abandoned. Several factors will influence the decision to stop the resuscitative effort. These will include the medical history and anticipated prognosis, the period between cardiac arrest and start of CPR, the interval to defibrillation and the period of advanced life support with continuing asystole and no reversible cause.

In many cases, particularly in out-of-hospital cardiac arrest, the underlying cause of arrest may be unknown or merely surmised and the decision is made to start resuscitation while further information is gathered. If it becomes clear that the underlying cause renders the situation futile, then resuscitation should be abandoned if the patient remains in asystole with all advanced life support measures in place. Information, such as an advance directive, can also become available, which makes discontinuation of the resuscitation attempt ethically correct.

In general, resuscitation should be continued as long as ventricular fibrillation persists. It is generally accepted that asystole for more than 20 min in the absence of a reversible cause, and with all advanced life support measures in place, is grounds for abandoning the resuscitation attempt.

In out-of-hospital cardiac arrest of cardiac origin, if recovery is going to occur, a return of spontaneous circulation is almost always established on site. Normothermic patients with primary cardiac arrest who require on-going CPR without any return of a pulse during transport to hospital almost never survive neurologically intact.

The decision to abandon the resuscitation attempt is made by the resuscitation team leader, but after consultation with the other team members. Ultimately, the decision is based on the clinical judgement that the patient's arrest is unresponsive to advanced life support.

## Decision making by non-physicians

Many cases of out-of-hospital cardiac arrest are attended by emergency medical technicians or paramedics, who face similar dilemmas about when resuscitation is futile and when it should be abandoned. In general, resuscitation is started in out-of-hospital cardiac arrest unless there is a valid advanced directive to the contrary or it is clear that resuscitation would be futile, for example, in cases of a mortal injury such as decapitation and hemicorporectomy, known prolonged submersion, incineration, rigor mortis, and dependent lividity. In such cases, the non-physician is recognising that death has occurred but is not certifying the cause of death (which can be done only by a physician or coroner in most countries).

But when should a decision be made to abandon a resuscitation attempt? Should paramedics trained in advanced life support be able to declare death when the patient remains in asystole after 20 min despite advanced life support techniques? In some countries, including the UK, paramedics may cease the resuscitation attempt in this situation. The strict protocol followed requires that certain conditions that might indicate a remote chance of survival (like hypothermia) are absent. The diagnosis of asystole must also be established beyond reasonable doubt and documented with ECG recordings.

Similar decisions about initiating resuscitation or recognising that death has occurred may have to be made by nurses in community nursing establishments for the aged or terminally ill. Hopefully, a decision on the merits of a resuscitation attempt will have been made before it is required and the matter of DNAR should always be addressed for every patient in these establishments.

## Mitigating circumstances

Certain circumstances, for example hypothermia at the time of cardiac arrest, will enhance the chances of recovery without neurological damage, and the normal prognostic criteria (such as asystole persisting for more than 20 min) are not applicable.

Sedative and analgesic drugs obscure the assessment of the level of consciousness in the patient who has a return of spontaneous circulation.

## Withdrawal of treatment after a resuscitation attempt

Prediction of the final neurological outcome in patients remaining comatose after regaining a spontaneous circulation is difficult during the first three days. There are no specific clinical signs that can predict outcome in the first few hours after the return of a spontaneous circulation. This topic is covered in more detail in Chapter 14.

## Key learning points

- Resuscitation should normally be started promptly and effectively, but we must recognise when these interventions are inappropriate and when they should cease.

## Further reading

Baskett PJF, Steen PA, Bossaert L. European Resuscitation Council Guidelines for Resuscitation 2005. Section 8. The ethics of resuscitation and end of life decisions. Resuscitation 2005;67 Suppl 1:S171-180.

Baskett PJ, Lim A. The varying ethical attitudes towards resuscitation in Europe. Resuscitation 2004;62:267-73.

Lemaire F, Bion J, Blanco J, et al. The European Union Directive on Clinical Research: present status of implementation in EU member states' legislations with regard to the incompetent patient. Intensive Care Med 2005;31:476-9.

Decisions relating to cardiopulmonary resuscitation. A joint statement from the BMA, RC(UK) and the RCN. March 2001

Nichol G, Huszti E, Rokosh J, Dumbrell A, McGowan J, Becker L. Impact of informed consent requirements on cardiac arrest research in the United States: exception from consent or from research? Resuscitation 2004;62:3-23.

ALS

# Supporting the Relative in Resuscitation Practice

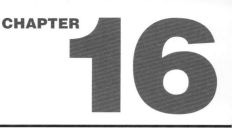

## CHAPTER 16

## Objectives

To understand:

▶ **How to support relatives witnessing attempted resuscitation.**

▶ **How to care for the recently bereaved.**

▶ **Religious and ethnic requirements when a patient has died.**

▶ **The legal and practical arrangements following a recent death.**

Throughout this chapter, the term 'relatives' includes close friends/significant others.

## Introduction

In many cases of out-of-hospital cardiac arrest, the person who performs CPR will be a close friend or relative. We recognise that there is a need to identify and respect relatives' wishes to remain with the patient.

Many relatives find it more distressing to be separated from their family member during these critical moments than to witness attempts at resuscitation. The preferences of patients and relatives should be taken into account by healthcare professionals, moving towards an ethic of more open clinical practice.

Relatives perceive a number of advantages of being present during resuscitation.

- It helps them come to terms with the reality of death, avoiding prolonged denial and contributing to a healthier bereavement.

- The relative can speak while there is still a chance that the dying person can hear.

- They are not distressed by being separated from a loved one when they feel the need to be present.

- They can see that everything possible was done for the dying person.

- They can touch and speak with the deceased whilst the body is warm.

There are potential disadvantages of relatives being present.

- The resuscitation attempt may prove distressing, particularly if the relatives are not kept informed.

- Relatives can physically, or emotionally, hinder the staff involved in the resuscitation attempt. Observed actions or remarks by medical or nursing staff may offend grieving family members.

- Relatives may be disturbed by the memory of events, although evidence indicates that fantasy is worse than fact. The staff should take into account the expectations of the bereaved and their cultural background during and following death.

- Relatives may demonstrate their emotions vocally or physically whilst others may wish to sit quietly or read religious text. The staff must have sufficient insight, knowledge and skills to anticipate these needs and identify potential problems.

## The involvement of relatives and friends

Care and consideration of the relative during resuscitation becomes increasingly important as procedures become more invasive. A member of the resuscitation team who is not actively involved in the attempt should escort any relatives wishing to be present during a resuscitation attempt. The following safeguards should be used:

- Acknowledge the difficulty of the situation. Ensure that they understand that they have a choice of whether or not to be present during resuscitation. Avoid provoking feelings of guilt whatever their decision.

- Explain that they will be looked after whether or not they enter the resuscitation room. Ensure that introductions are made and names are known.

- Give a clear explanation of what has happened in terms of the illness or injury and what they can expect to see when they enter the room.

- Ensure that the relatives understand that they will be able to leave and return at any time, and will always be accompanied.

- Ask the relative not to interfere with the resuscitation process but offer them the opportunity to touch the patient when they are told that it is safe to do so.

- Explain the procedures in simple terms. Ultimately, this may mean explaining that the resuscitation attempt has been unsuccessful and will be stopped.

If the patient dies, advise the relatives that there may be a brief interval while equipment is removed, after which they can return to be together in private. Under some circumstances, the coroner may require certain tubes to be left in place. Offer the relatives time to think about what has happened and the opportunity for further questions.

Hospitals should develop policies to suit their own environment to enable relatives to observe the attempted resuscitation of their loved one.

# Caring for the recently bereaved

Caring for the bereaved compassionately will ease the grieving process. Adapt the following considerations to the individual family and their cultural needs:

- early contact with one person, usually a nurse;

- provision of a suitable relatives' room;

- breaking bad news sympathetically and supporting the grief response appropriately;

- arranging for relatives to view the body;

- religious and pastoral care requirements;

- legal and practical arrangements;

- follow up and team support.

## Early contact with one person

Ideally this should be the person who has supported the relatives during the resuscitation attempt. If the resuscitation attempt was not observed allocate a member of the care team specifically to support the relatives. Communication between the emergency services and the receiving hospital should ensure that the arrival of relatives is anticipated. A warm, friendly and confident greeting will help to establish an open and honest relationship.

## Provision of a suitable room

This should provide the appropriate ambiance, space and privacy for relatives to ask questions and to express their emotions freely.

## Breaking bad news and supporting the grief response

An uncomplicated and honest approach will help avoid mixed messages. The breaking of bad news should be undertaken by the most appropriate person; this may not necessarily be a doctor. It may be more appropriate for the nurse who has been accompanying the relatives to break the news, although relatives may take comfort from talking to a doctor as well and this opportunity should always be offered. When preparing to talk to the relatives, consider the following:

- Prepare yourself mentally and physically. Check your clothing for blood, wash your hands and tidy your clothing.

- Confirm that you are talking with the correct relatives and establish their relationship to the deceased. Establish what they know and use this as the basis for your communication with them.

- Use tone of voice and non-verbal behaviour to support what you are saying. Smiles, nods, eye contact, the use of touch, facial expression and gestures can help support verbal communication.

- Use simple words and avoid medical jargon and platitudes that will be meaningless to the relative.

- Sit or position yourself next to the relative so that you are on the same level.

- Do not enter into a long preamble or question the relative about issues such as premorbid health. They want to know immediately whether their loved one is alive or dead.

- Introduce the word "dead", "died" or "death" at the earliest moment and reinforce this on at least one further occasion, so that there is no ambiguity.

- After breaking the news, do not be afraid to allow a period of silence while the facts are absorbed.

- Anticipate the different types of reaction/emotional response you may experience after breaking the bad news.

Possible responses to grief include:

- acute emotional distress/shock;

- anger;

- denial/disbelief;

- guilt;

- catatony.

These stages are not linear and individuals may move from one to another, returning to some repeatedly. An individual's gender, age and cultural background will influence the response to grief.

Respect cultural requirements and, where possible, provide written guidelines for individual ethnic minority groups.

## Arranging viewing of the body

Give relatives the opportunity to view the body. Advise relatives what to expect before viewing the body. People are less concerned about medical devices and equipment than staff believe. If the deceased has mutilating injuries, warn the relatives. Being in the physical presence of their loved one will help them work through the grieving process. Ensure the opportunity to touch/hold the deceased is given. Relatives should be accompanied by staff during the viewing process and they should remain near by to offer support or provide information as required.

## Religious requirements, legal and practical arrangements

Variations in handling the body and expressions of grief are influenced by the patient's religious convictions. Religious representatives from the patient's denomination or faith are usually available to attend in hospital. Hospital chaplains are a great source of strength and information to families and staff. Prayers, blessings, religious acts and procedure are all important in ensuring that relatives are not distressed further.

ALS

Legal and practical arrangements are equally important. These include:

- notification of the coroner or other appropriate authority;

- notification of the patient's family doctor;

- organ donation decisions;

- provision of information about what to do in the event of death;

- involvement of religious ministers;

- adhere to hospital procedure in the return of patients property and valuables;

- information concerning the social services that are available;

- information concerning post mortem examination where indicated;

- follow up arrangements, which may involve long-term counselling;

- provision of a telephone contact number for relatives to use and a named staff member who they can call should they have any further questions.

## Staff support and debriefing

Where and when possible, make arrangements for staff to discuss with the team leader and the rest of the team issues that emerged from the resuscitation event. This is an extremely powerful educational tool.

### Key learning points

- Many relatives want the opportunity to be present during the attempted resuscitation of their loved one. This may help the grieving process.

- Communication with bereaved relatives should be honest, simple, and supportive.

## Further reading

Adams S, Whitlock M, Bloomfield P, Baskett PJF. Should relatives watch resuscitation? BMJ 1994;308:1687-9.

Axelsson A, Zettergren M, Axelsson C. Good and bad experiences of family presence during acute care and resuscitation. What makes the difference? Eur J Cardiovasc Nurs 2005;4:161-9.

Kent H, McDowell J. Sudden bereavement in acute care settings. Nursing Standard 2004;19:6.

McLauchlan CAJ. Handling distressed relatives & breaking bad news. In: Driscoll P, Skinner D, Earlam R (editors) ABC of Major Trauma Third Edition. London, BMJ Books, 2000.

Royal College of Nursing. Witnessing Resuscitation: Guidance for Nursing staff. Royal College of Nursing, London, April 2002

Resuscitation Council (UK). Should relatives witness resuscitation? London, Resuscitation Council (UK), 1996.

ALS

ALS

# Audit and Outcome after Cardiac Arrest

## CHAPTER 17

## Objectives

To understand:

▶ **The reasons for the apparent variation in success rates following resuscitation.**

▶ **Why there is a need to adopt uniform reporting of outcome after cardiac arrest.**

▶ **What data need to be collected.**

▶ **How to collect the data.**

## Variability in outcome after cardiac arrest

Survival from out-of-hospital cardiac arrest varies substantially between health care systems. A review of emergency medical services (EMS) with a defibrillation capability that included 33,124 patients, reported a median survival to hospital discharge rate of 6.4% with a range of 0-20.7%. Summary data from 37 communities in Europe indicate that survival to hospital discharge after EMS-treated out-of-hospital cardiorespiratory arrest is 10.7%.

After in-hospital cardiac arrest, the reported survival to 24 h ranges from 13-59% and survival to discharge from 3-27%. The median survival to discharge after in-hospital cardiac arrest is around 15%. There are probably two main reasons for such variation; firstly, there are many confounders that influence outcome following cardiac arrest. These include:

- differences in the type of EMS system (e.g., availability of defibrillators, differences in response intervals);

- differences in the incidence of bystander CPR;

- different patient populations (e.g., a study may be confined to in-hospital cardiac arrests or may include pre-hospital arrests);

- the prevalence of co-morbid conditions;

- the frequency of implementing do-not-attempt-resuscitation (DNAR) policies;

- the primary arrest rhythm;

- the definition of cardiac arrest (e.g., inclusion of primary respiratory arrests);

- availability of cardiac arrest and medical emergency teams.

Secondly, there is lack of uniformity in reporting both the process and results of resuscitation attempts; for example, the definition of survival is reported variously as return of spontaneous circulation, or survival at 5 min, 1 h, 24 h, or to discharge from hospital. The lack of uniformity in cardiac arrest reporting makes it difficult to evaluate the impact on survival of individual factors, such as new drugs or techniques.

New interventions that improve survival rate only slightly are important because of the many victims of cardiac arrest each year. Local hospitals or healthcare systems are unlikely to have sufficient patients to identify these effects or eliminate confounders. One way around this dilemma is by adopting uniform definitions and collecting standardised data on both the process and outcome of resuscitation on large numbers of patients in multiple centres. Changes in the resuscitation process can then be introduced and evaluated using a reliable measure of outcome. This methodology enables drugs and techniques developed in experimental studies to be evaluated reliably in the clinical setting.

## Guidelines for uniform reporting of data following cardiac arrest: the Utstein style

In 1991 and 1997, representatives of the American Heart Association, the European Resuscitation Council, the Heart and Stroke Foundation of Canada, and the Australian Resuscitation Council produced guidelines for the uniform reporting of data for out-of-hospital and in-hospital cardiac arrest respectively. These were named the Utstein Guidelines after Utstein Abbey, near Stavanger, Norway, where the groups met. Key features of these guidelines were clear and precise definitions of interventions, intervals and outcomes, and the production of templates for reporting of resuscitation attempts. Despite standardising resuscitation terminology successfully, there were two main problems: it was difficult to capture many of the data items accurately (e.g., time of collapse) and the focus was on victims of ventricular fibrillation. In 2002, an International Liaison Committee on Resuscitation (ILCOR) task force reviewed the Utstein definitions and templates and in 2004 published a revised version in, which included:

- identification of 29 core data elements regarded as the minimum required for audit and quality improvement;

- revised and updated definitions of the core data elements;

- identification of supplementary data required for resuscitation research;

- identification of core time points and intervals to be collected and recorded;

- revised cardiac arrest data collection form;

- revised recording template for core data elements.

These covered out-of-hospital and in-hospital cardiac arrest in both adults and children.

## Core data elements defined in the 2004 Utstein template

The 29 core data elements defined in alphabetical order are listed in Table 17.1. For the precise definitions consult the appropriate publication.

| |
|---|
| Arrest, witnessed |
| Assisted ventilation |
| Attempted defibrillation |
| Bystander CPR |
| Cardiac arrest |
| Cause of arrest/aetiology |
| Chest compressions |
| CPR |
| Date of arrest |
| Date of birth/age |
| Date of discharge/death |
| Defibrillation attempt before EMS arrival |
| Drugs |
| Emergency Medical Services (EMS) |
| End of event |
| First monitored rhythm |
| Location of arrest |
| Neurological outcome at discharge from hospital |
| Patient identification |
| Resuscitation |
| Resuscitation attempted by EMS personnel |
| Resuscitation not attempted by EMS personnel |
| Return of spontaneous circulation |
| Sex |
| Shockable or non-shockable rhythm |
| Successful CPR before EMS arrival |
| Survived event |
| Survival to hospital discharge |
| Sustained return of spontaneous circulation |

**Table 17.1 Core data items in the 2004 Utstein template**

## Core time points and intervals

Although some time intervals are known to be key determinants of successful outcome (e.g., collapse to first shock in VF), collection of these data is often difficult and inaccurate because of factors such as the urgency of the situation and the use of unsynchronised clocks. Consequently, in the revised guidelines the number of core time points has been reduced significantly:

- time of witnessed or monitored arrest;
- time call received;
  - by EMS operator;
  - resuscitation team summoned;
- time of first rhythm analysis or assessment of need for CPR;
- time of first CPR attempts;
- time of first defibrillation attempt if shockable rhythm;
- date of death.

Several supplementary times are defined, recognising that although they probably are relatively unimportant in terms of outcome, they may be used as indicators of quality assurance:

- time first emergency vehicle is mobile;
- time vehicle stops;
- time of return of spontaneous circulation;
- time vascular access achieved and drugs given;
- time CPR stopped/time of death.

## Post-resuscitation care

It is now widely recognised that the quality of treatment in the post-resuscitation phase is a significant determinant of outcome. Many intensive care units collect comprehensive data on all admissions, including survivors of cardiac arrest. An Utstein style template has been defined recently in an attempt to standardise the way in which data are defined and collected in the post-resuscitation phase. This should enable meaningful comparison between centres and may help to determine the impact on outcome of different treatment strategies (e.g., therapeutic hypothermia).

## How do we collect the data?

Having defined clearly the core processes and outcomes that will enable the effects of changes in the treatment of cardiac arrest to be studied, a method for collecting these data is required. The data on outcome following cardiac arrest can be entered into individual cardiac arrest reports and into a cardiac arrest registry.

ALS

# Cardiac Arrest Data Collection Form

Date of arrest        YYYY/MM/DD

Patient identifier    [        ]    (first name, last name, or ID number)

**Sex**               [        ]

Age    [        ] years (estimated)        OR        Date of birth    YYYY/MM/DD

Cardiac arrest determined by    [        ]

Cause of arrest    [        ]

Treatment before EMS arrival

| | |
|---|---|
| Bystander CPR | [        ] |
| Defibrillation by bystander ☐ or implanted defibrillator ☐ | |

Resuscitation attempted by EMS

Location of arrest        out of hospital [        ]        in hospital [        ]

Witnessed        [        ]        If witnessed, time of arrest    hh:mm

Initial rhythm        [        ]

Chest compressions    [        ]

Defibrillation attempt    [        ]

Ventilation        [        ]        Drugs [        ] [        ] [        ]


Time of collapse        hh:mm (estimated)

Time of call receipt        hh:mm

Time vehicle stopped        hh:mm

Time of first rhythm analysis        hh:mm


Spontaneous circulation on arrival in ED        [        ]

Hospital admission        [        ]

Hospital discharge        [        ]

Date of hospital discharge (or death)        YYYY/MM/DD

Neurological status at discharge (CPC)        [        ]

**Figure 17.1 The 2004 Utstein-style cardiac arrest data collection form**

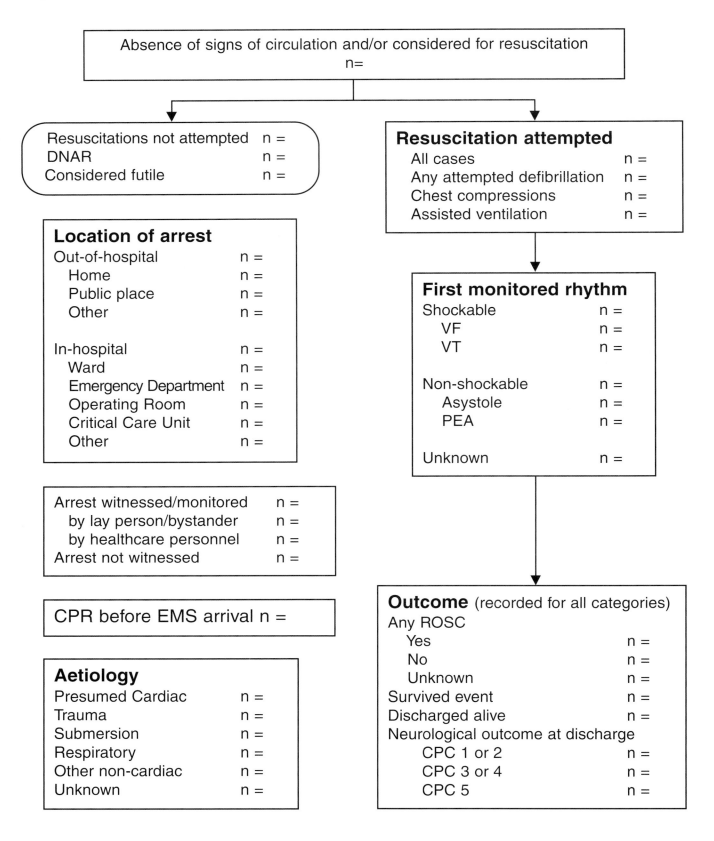

**Figure 17.2 The 2004 Utstein template for recording cardiac arrest data**

## Cardiac arrest report

Core data elements for each cardiac arrest resuscitation attempt are recorded manually and/or electronically. The data should be easy to collect, reliable and include patient, process and outcome elements. By collecting core data using the definitions described above, comparisons can be made not only within, but also between hospitals, locally, nationally and internationally. A simplified standardised data collection form is shown in Figure 17.1. When new techniques or drugs are being investigated, specific research forms may be required but these should still include core data points defined in the Utstein template.

## Cardiac arrest registry

Previously, separate templates or registries were used for out-of-hospital and in-hospital cardiac arrests. They included both essential and desirable data points and concentrated on patients who had suffered a VF arrest. These have now been replaced with a single template that records only core data. All initial arrest rhythms are included but the capability for separate analysis of VF arrests is retained. Because the registry contains details of many arrests, it is generally a tool that is used to monitor the effect of changes in practice or to identify areas that require improvement. The Utstein reporting template for this process is shown in Figure 17.2.

No single form will meet with global approval. Hospitals and EMS systems with an established report form will be reluctant to change. If unwilling to adopt the styles described above, hospitals and EMS systems are encouraged strongly to incorporate the core Utstein variables into their individual reporting forms.

## Key learning points

- Attempts to improve cardiopulmonary resuscitation are hindered by lack of uniform definitions and inconsistent reporting of the process and outcome.

- Inconsistency in reporting makes it impossible to compare results from different studies and healthcare systems reliably.

- The science of resuscitation will be enhanced by defining the essential variables to be collected and by adopting a uniform reporting system.

## Further reading

Atwood C, Eisenberg MS, Herlitz J, Rea TD. Incidence of EMS-treated out-of-hospital cardiac arrest in Europe. Resuscitation 2005;67:75-80.

Gabbott D, Smith G, Mitchell M, Colquhoun M, Nolan J, Soar J, Pitcher D, Perkins G, Phillips B, King B, Spearpoint K. Cardiopulmonary resuscitation standards for clinical practice and training in the UK. Resuscitation 2005; 64: 13-19.

Gwinnutt CL, Columb M, Harris R. Outcome after cardiac arrest in adults in UK hospitals: effect of the 1997 guidelines. Resuscitation 2000;47:125-36.

Jacobs I, Nadkarni V, Bahr J, et al. Cardiac arrest and cardiopulmonary resuscitation outcome reports: update and simplification of the Utstein templates for resuscitation registries. A statement for healthcare professionals from a task force of the International Liaison Committee on Resuscitation. Resuscitation 2004;63:233-49.

Langhelle A, Nolan J, Herlitz J, et al. Recommended guidelines for reviewing, reporting, and conducting research on post-resuscitation care: The Utstein style. Resuscitation 2005;66:271-83.

Nichol G, Stiell IG, Laupacis A, De Maio VJ, Wells GA. A cumulative meta-analysis of the effectiveness of defibrillator-capable emergency medical services for victims of out-of-hospital cardiac arrest. Ann Emerg Med 1999;34:517-25.

Pell JP, Sirel JM, Marsden AK, Ford I, Walker NL, Cobbe SM. Presentation, management, and outcome of out of hospital cardiopulmonary arrest: comparison by underlying aetiology. Heart 2003;89:839-42.

Tunstall-Pedoe H, Bailey L, Chamberlain DA, Marsden AK, Ward ME, Zideman DA. Survey of 3765 cardiopulmonary resuscitations in British hospitals (the BRESUS study): methods and overall results. BMJ 1992;304:1347-51.

ALS

# Appendix 1. Lay Rescuer Basic Life Support

## Introduction

This section contains the guidelines for out-of-hospital, single lay rescuer, adult basic life support (BLS). Basic life support implies that no equipment is employed other than a protective device.

It is well documented that interruptions in chest compression are common and are associated with a reduced chance of survival for the victim. The 'perfect' solution is to deliver continuous compressions whilst giving ventilations independently. This is possible when the victim has an advanced airway in place, and is discussed in Chapters 5 and 6. Chest-compression-only CPR is another way to increase the number of compressions given and will, by definition, eliminate pauses. It is effective for a limited period only (about 5 min) and is not recommended as standard management of out-of-hospital cardiac arrest.

The following changes in the BLS guidelines have been made to reflect the greater importance placed on chest compression, and to attempt to reduce the number and duration of pauses:

1) The diagnosis of cardiac arrest is made if a victim is unresponsive and not breathing normally.

2) Teach rescuers to place their hands on the centre of the chest, rather than to spend more time using the 'rib margin' method.

3) Give each rescue breath over 1 sec rather than 2 sec.

4) Use a ratio of compressions to ventilations is 30:2 for all adult victims of sudden cardiac arrest (SCA). This same ratio is used for children when attended by a lay rescuer.

5) For an adult victim, omit the initial 2 rescue breaths and give 30 compressions immediately after cardiac arrest is established.

To aid teaching and learning, the sequence of actions has been simplified. In some cases, simplification has been based on recently published evidence; in others there was no evidence that the previous, more complicated, sequence had any beneficial effect on survival.

There are other changes in the guidelines. In particular, allowance has been made for the rescuer who is unable or unwilling to perform rescue breathing. It is well recorded that reluctance to perform mouth-to-mouth ventilation, in spite of the lack of evidence of risk, inhibits many would-be rescuers from attempting any form of resuscitation. These guidelines encourage chest compression alone in such circumstances.

The guidelines 2000 introduced the concept of checking for 'signs of a circulation'. This change was made because of the evidence that relying on a check of the carotid pulse to diagnose cardiac arrest is unreliable and time consuming, mainly, but not exclusively, when attempted by non-healthcare professionals. Subsequent studies have shown that checking for breathing is also prone to error, particularly as agonal gasps are frequently misdiagnosed as normal breathing. In Guidelines 2005 the absence of breathing, in a non-responsive victim, continues to be the main sign of cardiac arrest. Also highlighted is the need to identify agonal gasps as another, positive, indication to start CPR.

Finally, there is recognition that delivering chest compressions is tiring. It is now recommended that, where more than one rescuer is present, another should take over the compressions (with a minimum of delay) about every 2 min to prevent fatigue and maintain the quality of performance.

## Adult BLS sequence

Basic life support consists of the following sequence of actions (Figure A1):

1 **Make sure the victim, any bystanders and you are safe.**

2 **Check the victim for a response.**

- Gently shake his shoulders and ask loudly, 'Are you all right?'

3 A **If he responds:**

- Leave him in the position in which you find him provided there is no further danger.

- Try to find out what is wrong with him and get help if needed.

- Reassess him regularly.

3 B **If he does not respond:**

- Shout for help.

- Turn the victim onto his back and then open the airway using head tilt and chin lift:

  - Place your hand on his forehead and gently tilt his head back.
  - With your fingertips under the point of the victim's chin, lift the chin to open the airway.

4 **Keeping the airway open, look, listen, and feel for normal breathing.**

- Look for chest movement.

- Listen at the victim's mouth for breath sounds.

- Feel for air on your cheek.

ALS

## Adult Basic Life Support

ALS

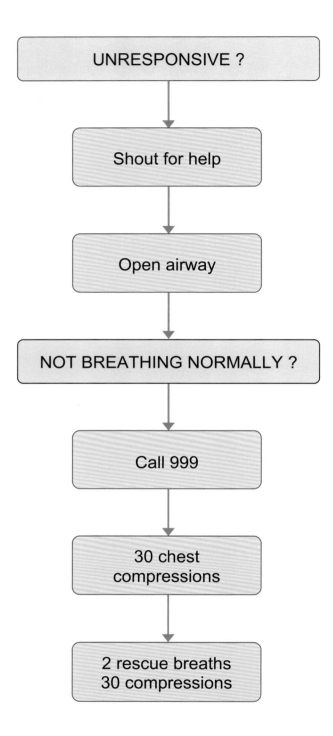

**Figure A1 Algorithm for lay rescuer basic life support**

ALS

In the first few minutes after cardiac arrest, a victim may be barely breathing, or taking infrequent, noisy, gasps. Do not confuse this with normal breathing.

Look, listen, and feel for **no more** than **10 sec** to determine if the victim is breathing normally. If you have any doubt whether breathing is normal, act as if it is **not** normal.

**5 A  If he is breathing normally:**

- Turn him into the recovery position (**see below**).

- Send or go for help, or call for an ambulance.

- Check for continued breathing.

**5 B  If he is not breathing normally:**

- Ask someone to call for an ambulance or, if you are on your own, do this yourself; you may need to leave the victim. Start chest compression as follows:

  - Kneel by the side of the victim.

  - Place the heel of one hand in the centre of the victim's chest.

  - Place the heel of your other hand on top of the first hand.

  - Interlock the fingers of your hands and ensure that pressure is not applied over the victim's ribs. Do not apply any pressure over the upper abdomen or the bottom end of the bony sternum (breastbone).

  - Position yourself vertically above the victim's chest and, with your arms straight, press down on the sternum 4 - 5 cm.

  - After each compression, release all the pressure on the chest without losing contact between your hands and the sternum. Repeat at a rate of about 100 times a minute (a little less than 2 compressions a second).

  - Compression and release should take an equal amount of time.

**6 A  Combine chest compression with rescue breaths.**

- After 30 compressions open the airway again using head tilt and chin lift.

- Pinch the soft part of the victim's nose closed, using the index finger and thumb of your hand on his forehead.

- Allow his mouth to open, but maintain chin lift.

- Take a normal breath and place your lips around his mouth, making sure that you have a good seal.

- Blow steadily into his mouth whilst watching for his chest to rise; take about one second to make his

chest rise as in normal breathing; this is an effective rescue breath.

- Maintaining head tilt and chin lift, take your mouth away from the victim and watch for his chest to fall as air comes out.

- Take another normal breath and blow into the victim's mouth once more to give a total of two effective rescue breaths. Then return your hands without delay to the correct position on the sternum and give a further 30 chest compressions.

- Continue with chest compressions and rescue breaths in a ratio of 30:2.

- Stop to recheck the victim only if he starts breathing **normally**; otherwise **do not interrupt resuscitation.**

If your rescue breaths do not make the chest rise as in normal breathing, then before your next attempt:

- Check the victim's mouth and remove any visible obstruction.

- Recheck that there is adequate head tilt and chin lift.

- Do not attempt more than 2 breaths each time before returning to chest compressions.

If there is more than one rescuer present, another should take over CPR about every 2 min to prevent fatigue. Ensure the minimum of delay during the changeover of rescuers.

**6 B  Chest-compression-only CPR.**

- If you are not able, or are unwilling, to give rescue breaths, give chest compressions only.

- If chest compressions only are given, these should be continuous at a rate of 100 a minute.

- Stop to recheck the victim only if he starts breathing **normally**; otherwise do not interrupt resuscitation.

**7  Continue resuscitation until:**

- qualified help arrives and takes over; or

- the victim starts breathing normally; or

- you become exhausted.

## Explanatory notes

### Risk to the rescuer

The safety of both the rescuer and victim are paramount during a resuscitation attempt. There have been few incidents of rescuers suffering adverse effects from undertaking CPR, with only isolated reports of infections such as tuberculosis (TB) and severe acute respiratory distress syndrome (SARS). Transmission of HIV during CPR has never been reported. There have been no human

ALS

studies to address the effectiveness of barrier devices during CPR; however, laboratory studies have shown that certain filters, or barrier devices with one-way valves, prevent oral bacteria transmission from the victim to the rescuer during mouth-to-mouth ventilation. Rescuers should take appropriate safety precautions where feasible, especially if the victim is known to have a serious infection, such as TB.

### Initial rescue breaths

During the first few minutes after non-asphyxial cardiac arrest the blood oxygen content remains high. Ventilation is, therefore, less important than chest compression at this time.

It is well recognised that skill acquisition and retention are aided by simplification of the BLS sequence of actions. It is also recognised that rescuers are frequently unwilling to carry out mouth-to-mouth ventilation for a variety of reasons, including fear of infection and distaste for the procedure. For these reasons, and to emphasise the priority of chest compressions, it is recommended that, in most adults, CPR should start with chest compressions rather than initial ventilations.

### Jaw thrust

The jaw thrust technique is not recommended for lay rescuers because it is difficult to learn and perform. Therefore, the lay rescuer should open the airway using a head-tilt-chin-lift manoeuvre.

### Agonal gasps

Agonal gasps are present in up to 40% of cardiac arrest victims. Laypeople should, therefore, be taught to begin CPR if the victim is unconscious (unresponsive) and not breathing normally. It should be emphasised during training that agonal gasps occur commonly in the first few minutes after SCA. They are an indication for starting CPR immediately and should not be confused with normal breathing.

### Mouth-to-nose ventilation

Mouth-to-nose ventilation is an effective alternative to mouth-to-mouth ventilation. It may be considered if the victim's mouth is seriously injured or cannot be opened, the rescuer is assisting a victim in the water, or a mouth-to-mouth seal is difficult to achieve.

### Mouth-to-tracheostomy ventilation

Mouth-to-tracheostomy ventilation may be used for a victim with a tracheostomy tube or tracheal stoma who requires rescue breathing.

### Bag-mask ventilation

Considerable practice and skill are required to use a bag and mask for ventilation. The lone rescuer has to be able to open the airway with a jaw thrust whilst simultaneously holding the mask to the victim's face. It is a technique that is appropriate only for lay rescuers who work in highly specialised areas, such as where there is a risk of cyanide poisoning or exposure to other toxic agents. There are other specific circumstances in which non-healthcare providers receive extended training in first aid which could include training, and retraining, in the use of bag-mask ventilation. The same strict training that applies to healthcare professionals should be followed and the two-person technique is preferable.

### Chest compression

In most circumstances it will be possible to identify the correct hand position for compression without removing the victim's clothes. If in any doubt, remove outer clothing.

In Guidelines 2000 a method was recommended for finding the correct hand position for chest compression by placing one finger on the lower end of the sternum and sliding the other hand down to it. It has been shown that the same hand position can be found more quickly if rescuers are taught to 'place the heel of your hand in the centre of the chest with the other hand on top', provided the teaching includes a demonstration of placing the hands in the middle of the lower half of the sternum.

Whilst performing chest compression:

a) Each time compressions are resumed, the rescuer should place his hands without delay 'in the centre of the chest'.

b) Compress the chest at a rate of about 100 a minute.

c) Pay attention to achieving the full compression depth of 4-5 cm (for an adult).

d) Allow the chest to recoil completely after each compression.

e) Take approximately the same amount of time for compression and relaxation.

f) Minimise interruptions in chest compression.

g) Do not rely on a palpable carotid or femoral pulse as a gauge of effective arterial flow.

h) 'Compression rate' refers to the speed at which compressions are given, not the total number delivered in each minute. The number delivered is determined not only by the rate, but also by the number of interruptions to open the airway, deliver rescue breaths, and allow AED analysis.

### Compression-only CPR

Studies have shown that chest-compression-only CPR may be as effective as combined ventilation and compression in the first few minutes after non-asphyxial arrest. Laypeople should, therefore, be encouraged to do compression-only CPR if they are unable or unwilling to provide rescue breaths, although combined chest compression and ventilation is the better method of CPR.

### Over-the-head CPR

Over-the-head CPR for a single rescuer and straddle CPR for two rescuers may be considered for resuscitation in confined spaces.

### Recovery position

There are several variations of the recovery position, each with its own advantages. No single position is perfect for all victims. The position should be stable, near a true lateral position with the head dependent, and with no pressure on the chest to impair breathing.

To place a victim in the recovery position:

- Remove the victim's spectacles.

- Kneel beside the victim and make sure that both his legs are straight.

- Place the arm nearest to you out at right angles to his body, elbow bent with the hand palm uppermost.

- Bring the far arm across the chest, and hold the back of the hand against the victim's cheek nearest to you.

- With your other hand, grasp the far leg just above the knee and pull it up, keeping the foot on the ground.

- Keeping the victim's hand pressed against his cheek, pull on the far leg to roll the victim towards you onto his side.

- Adjust the upper leg so that both the hip and knee are bent at right angles.

- Tilt the head back to make sure the airway remains open.

- Adjust the hand under the cheek, if necessary, to keep the head tilted.

- Check breathing regularly.

If the victim has to be kept in the recovery position for **more than 30 min** turn him to the opposite side to relieve the pressure on the lower arm.

## Choking

### Recognition

Because recognition of choking (airway obstruction by a foreign body) is the key to successful outcome, it is important not to confuse this emergency with fainting, heart attack, seizure or other conditions that may cause sudden respiratory distress, cyanosis, or loss of consciousness.

Foreign bodies may cause either mild or severe airway obstruction. The signs and symptoms enabling differentiation between mild and severe airway obstruction are summarised in the table below. It is important to ask the conscious victim 'Are you choking?'

| General signs of choking | |
|---|---|
| • Attack occurs while eating<br>• Victim may clutch his neck | |

| Signs of mild airway obstruction | Signs of severe airway obstruction |
|---|---|
| *Response to question 'Are you choking?'*<br>• Victim speaks and answers yes<br><br>*Other signs*<br>• Victim is able to speak, cough and breathe | *Response to question 'Are you choking?'*<br>• Victim unable to speak<br>• Victim may respond by nodding<br>*Other signs*<br>• Victim unable to breathe<br>• Breathing sounds wheezy<br>• Attempts at coughing are silent<br>• Victim may be unconscious |

### Adult choking sequence

(This sequence is also suitable for use in children over the age of 1 year)

**1   If the victim shows signs of mild airway obstruction:**

Encourage him to continue coughing, but do nothing else.

**2   If the victim shows signs of severe airway obstruction and is conscious:**

- Give up to five back slaps.

  - Stand to the side and slightly behind the victim.

  - Support the chest with one hand and lean the victim well forwards so that when the obstructing object is dislodged it comes out of the mouth rather than goes further down the airway.

  - Give **up to** five sharp slaps between the shoulder blades with the heel of your other hand.

- Check to see if each back slap has relieved the airway obstruction. The aim is to relieve the obstruction with each slap rather than necessarily to give all five.

- If five back slaps fail to relieve the airway obstruction give up to five abdominal thrusts.

  - Stand behind the victim and put both arms round the upper part of his abdomen.

  - Lean the victim forwards.

  - Clench your fist and place it between the umbilicus (navel) and the bottom end of the sternum (breastbone).

  - Grasp this hand with your other hand and pull sharply inwards and upwards.

ALS

- Repeat up to five times.

- If the obstruction is still not relieved, continue alternating five back slaps with five abdominal thrusts.

**3   If the victim becomes unconscious:**

- Support the victim carefully to the ground.

- Immediately call an ambulance.

- Begin CPR (from 5B of the Adult BLS Sequence). Healthcare providers, trained and experienced in feeling for a carotid pulse, should initiate chest compressions even if a pulse is present in the unconscious choking victim.

### Explanatory notes

Following successful treatment for choking, foreign material may nevertheless remain in the upper or lower respiratory tract and cause complications later.  Victims with a persistent cough, difficulty swallowing, or with the sensation of an object being still stuck in the throat should therefore be referred for a medical opinion.

Abdominal thrusts can cause serious internal injuries and all victims receiving abdominal thrusts should be examined for injury by a doctor.

## Resuscitation of children and victims of drowning

Both ventilation and compression are important for victims of cardiac arrest when the oxygen stores become depleted - about 4-6 min after collapse from ventricular fibrillation (VF) and immediately after collapse for victims of asphyxial arrest.  Previous guidelines tried to take into account the difference in causation, and recommended that victims of identifiable asphyxia (drowning; trauma; intoxication) and children should receive 1 min of CPR before the lone rescuer left the victim to get help.  The majority of cases of sudden cardiac arrest out of hospital, however, occur in adults and are of cardiac origin due to VF. These additional recommendations, therefore, added to the complexity of the guidelines whilst affecting only a minority of victims.

Also important is that many children do not receive resuscitation because potential rescuers fear causing harm. This fear is unfounded; it is far better to use the adult BLS sequence for resuscitation of a child than to do nothing.

For ease of teaching and retention, therefore, laypeople should be taught that the adult sequence may also be used for children who are not responsive and not breathing.

The following minor modifications to the adult sequence will, however, make it even more suitable for use in children:

- Give five initial rescue breaths before starting chest compressions (adult sequence of actions 5B).

- A lone rescuer should perform CPR for approximately 1 min before going for help.

- Compress the chest by approximately one-third of its depth. Use two fingers for an infant under 1 year; use one or two hands for a child over 1 year as needed to achieve an adequate depth of compression.

The same modifications of five initial breaths, and 1 min of CPR by the lone rescuer before getting help, may improve outcome for victims of drowning. This modification should be taught only to those who have a specific duty of care to potential drowning victims (e.g., lifeguards).

Drowning is easily identified.  It can be difficult, on the other hand, for a layperson to determine whether cardiorespiratory arrest has been caused by trauma or intoxication.  These victims should, therefore, be managed according to the standard protocol.

## Further reading

International Liaison Committee on Resuscitation. Part 2. Adult Basic Life Support. 2005 International Consensus on Cardiopulmonary Resuscitation and Emergency Cardiovascular Care Science with Treatment Recommendations. Resuscitation 2005;67:187-201.

Handley AJ, Koster R, Monsieurs K, Perkins GD, Davies S, Bossaert L. European Resuscitation Council Guidelines for Resuscitation 2005.Section 2 Adult basic life support and use of automated external defibrillators. Resuscitation 2005; 67 Suppl 1:S7-23.

# Appendix 2. Useful Websites

| | |
|---|---|
| **www.resus.org.uk** | Resuscitation Council UK |
| **www.erc.edu** | European Resuscitation Council |
| **www.c2005.org** | 2005 International Consensus on CPR and ECC Science with Treatment Recommendations |
| **www.bcs.com** | British Cardiac Society |
| **www.escardio.org** | European Society of Cardiology |
| **www.amercianheart.org** | American Heart Association |
| **www.ics.ac.uk** | Intensive Care Society |
| **www.esicm.org** | European Society of Intensive Care Medicine |
| **www.aagbi.org** | Association of Anaesthetists of Great Britain and Ireland |
| **www.cochrane.org** | Cochrane Collaboration |
| **www.bestbets.org** | Best evidence topics in emergency medicine |
| **www.eaaci.net** | The European Academy of Allergology and Clinical Immunology |

ALS

# NOTES

ALS

# NOTES

ALS

# NOTES

# NOTES

ALS